Student Study Guide

to accompany

Exercise Physiology
Theory and Application to Fitness and Performance
third edition

Scott K. Powers
University of Florida

Edward T. Howley
University of Tennessee-Knoxville

Prepared by

Jeff Coombes-University of Florida
Louise Fletcher-University of Florida
Lou D. Powers-University of Florida
Scott K. Powers
Edward T. Howley

A1013789

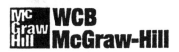

Boston, Massachusetts Burr Ridge, Illinois Dubuque, Iowa
Madison, Wisconsin New York, New York San Francisco, California St. Louis, Missouri

WCB/McGraw-Hill

A Division of The McGraw-Hill Companies

ISBN 0-697-29518-4

Printed in the United States of America

67890 QPD 09

Table of contents

Preface

This workbook is designed to accompany the textbook *Exercise Physiology: Theory and Application to Fitness and Performance* by Powers and Howley. The purpose of this study guide is twofold: 1) to improve your study and test-taking skills, and 2) to provide sets of structured learning activities that correspond to the textbook chapters.

The first section of this book, entitled *Student Study Strategies*, contains a list of proven study techniques. Even the most accomplished student will find one or more tips that will prove useful in understanding and retention of important concepts.

The remainder of this book is a series of structured learning modules that correspond to each chapter of the textbook. Each module lists the major learning objectives of a chapter and provides detailed multiple choice, true-false, and matching exams. These practice exams are designed to be comprehensive and cover the chapter learning objectives as well as all of the key terms covered in the chapter. An answer section at the end of each exam contains the correct answers to questions.

Student Success Strategies

Are you a "fast starter" but "slow finisher" when it comes to attending and preparing for your classes each semester? In other words, do you start the term like a ball of fire and then fade after a few weeks? While this is not uncommon, there are some fundamental strategies that can maximize your chances of getting the most from each class and increase your "academic endurance". This guide will introduce you to some of these strategies and provide you with a list of learning objectives and sample test questions for each chapter contained in the text, *Exercise Physiology: Theory and application to fitness and performance* by Powers and Howley.

Success Strategy #1

Establish goals

Imagine for a minute that you were asked to run a race without a finish line. You are probably saying "that's ridiculous!" You're right! And trying to accomplish anything in college or in life is just as difficult if you don't have goals to work toward. Goals can be academic (i.e. grades), personal (i.e. fitness) and other forms of self-improvement. It is important to have both short-term and long term goals, keeping in mind the following:
- Establish goals that are specific, realistic, and measurable.
- Goals should be written down, not just in your mind.
- Keep goals posted somewhere that you'll see them daily.
- Re-evaluate your goals periodically.
- Reward yourself for accomplishment of your goals.

Success Strategy #2

Manage your time wisely

Good time management is critical for success in both college and career. A daily "to-do" list and a weekly or monthly planner help you stay on track. Identify your greatest time-wasters and begin to examine ways to reduce them. Some basic time scheduling principles include:
- Avoid marathon study sessions. Study in blocks of one hour with ten minute breaks.
- Utilize daytime hours for tasks which require great concentration.
- Evaluate the time needed for each course you're taking. A general rule of thumb is: 2 hours outside class for every 1 hour in class. (ex. 3 credit hour class = 6 hours outside class per week)
- Schedule time immediately after class to edit and review notes.
- Schedule time just before class to review notes and assigned readings.
- Schedule continual review of previously learned material, not just new material.

Good time management begins with proper scheduling but also includes the following principles:
- Learn to say "no" to those activities and people that prevent you from achieving your goals.
- Don't try to do everything yourself. Delegate responsibilities to others.
- Schedule time for yourself everyday and don't feel guilty.
- Take breaks to improve your overall productivity.
- Eat well-balanced meals and get plenty of rest and exercise.
- Double your time estimates for assignments and start well in advance of due dates.

Success Strategy #3

Attend class regularly

Regular class attendance is essential since your textbook is a "supplement" to your classroom lecture material, not a "substitute". In addition, researchers have shown that many students learn best through active participation in class discussions. Even if your class is a large lecture format, you can keep mentally alert by listening for answers to potential test questions such as those provided in this guide as well as asking questions for clarification of points that are not completely understood.

Success Strategy #4

Determine your learning style

There are numerous theories about learning, but the most important thing is to determine how you learn best and adapt your study regime to enhance your preferred style. Ask yourself the following questions:
- Do I learn best by getting involved in class discussions?
- Do I learn best by sitting and listening?
- Do I learn best by understanding the broad concepts and then filling in the details?
- Do I learn best by figuring things out myself through laboratory experiences?

Once you have analyzed the way you learn best, consider changing your approach to classroom behavior and studying outside the classroom. For example, if you know that you learn best by active involvement, ask relevant questions in class, get to know your instructor, and form discussion groups with other class members.

Success Strategy #5

Take systematic lecture notes

Take lecture notes in a systematic manner that will make exam review easier. The following principles should be kept in mind:
- Date and identify each set of notes.
- Do not try to take "word-for-word" notes.
- Use your own words except for scientific vocabulary, formulas, etc.
- Copy diagrams, examples.
- Record instructor's emphasized points.
- Leave space in notes for later clarification.
- Use a modified outline form.
- Develop your own shorthand only if recognizable later.
- Review and edit notes immediately after class.

While you may already have a system of note-taking which works well, consider a system that was developed at Cornell University and has been used successfully by college students for over 40 years[0]. The Cornell System of taking notes not only provides a systematic method but also provides a "built-in" study system for examination review. The only special equipment needed is:
- a 3-ring binder
- loose-leaf notebook paper with a vertical line drawn down the left-hand side of the page approximately 2, or 2 1/2 inches over

---

[0] Pauk, Walter. How to Study in College. 1989, Boston, Houghton Mifflin Co.

and a horizontal line drawn approximately 2 inches across at
the bottom of the page

Using the basic note-taking principles listed above, record your notes as follows using only one
side of the paper.
- Record your notes in the right-hand column.
- Reduce the notes to key words, phrases or questions to use as
  recall devices when studying. Record these in the left-hand
  column.
- As you study, cover-up the right-hand column of your notes and recall
  the information from the lecture notes.
- Check for accuracy.
- Continue to review and recite periodically throughout the term
  to combat forgetting.
- Use the space at the bottom of the page for summarizing your
  notes to be sure you understand the material and aren't just
  memorizing information.

On the following page, we provide an exercise physiology example (Chapter 2 - Control of
Internal Environment) of how to use the Cornell System of note-taking:

Control of Internal Environment

How do the terms homeostasis & steady state differ?

① homeostasis - constant & normal internal environment

② steady state - constant but not always normal internal environment
(example: elevated body temp. during long run)

Identify & define 3 components of biological control system.

③ components of biological control systems
- receptor: change detector
- integrating center: signal receiver
                              control box
- effector: corrects disturbance
(example: control of arterial blood pressure

arterial blood pressure (110, 105, 100, 95) vs time (0 1 2 3 4 5 6 7 8)
average arterial pressure

The body has hundreds of control systems.
Each is designed to help the body maintain homeostasis or a normal internal environment
The components of a biological control system are:
① receptor ② integrating center and ③ effector

You may want to use the back of your notebook paper to create visual diagrams illustrating the written material. These "mind maps" use yet another one of your senses to increase your learning potential.

Success Strategy #6

Read to understand

Textbook reading is more that starting on page one and reading until you reach the end of the chapter. Just as you usually "preview" a movie before you decide to go and see it, textbook reading should begin by previewing the chapter.
- Read the introduction, look at chapter headings and key words.
- Examine the learning objectives provided and then as you read you are reading with a purpose--to achieve these objectives.
- Do not "highlight" as you read. Read a section and then go back and highlight after you've identified the main ideas.
- After reading each chapter, state or recite (out loud) in your own words the important points to ensure a good understanding, not just memorization.
- Finally, test yourself on the chapter using the sample questions provided in this guide.

Success Strategy #7

Exam preparation begins on the first day of class

While exam preparation is really the culmination of everything we've been discussing (time management, class attendance, good note-taking, textbook reading), when it is time to formally prepare for the exam there are certain things to think about.

First, are you preparing for an objective (multiple choice, matching, fill-in-the-blank, short answer) or an essay exam? Objective exams are common in Exercise Physiology classes due to the nature of the material and size of classes. An objective exam consisting of mostly multiple choice questions requires recognition of correct answers whereas an essay exam requires recall of detailed information, organization, and drawing conclusions.

At least one week before the exam, consolidate lecture notes and textbook notes, handouts, quizzes etc. You are accomplishing several things as you complete this consolidation process: 1) beginning the review process, 2) categorizing information to assist in retrieving from your memory, and 3) preparing a condensed set of notes that you can use as a refresher immediately prior to the exam. Make 3 x 5 cards to carry around with you. Utilize study groups. Give yourself a timed exam using some of the questions in this guide with the approximate number of questions you'll have on the exam.

Success Strategy #8

Regard test taking as an opportunity, not an obstacle

Do any of the following statements sound familiar?
- I knew the material but the instructor asked "trick" questions.
- I studied all the "wrong" things.
- I've learned the "most" from the classes in which I've gotten the worst grades.

Unfortunately, exams do provoke a certain amount of stress and do not always accurately reflect what you've learned. But, the following principles kept in mind on exam day should increase your chances of a test becoming an opportunity, not an obstacle.
- First and foremost, be prepared.
- Read all instructions carefully.
- Assess the amount of time you should allow for each question.
- Don't spend too much time on any one question.
- Put a check mark by questions which can't be quickly answered and return if time allows.
- Try to stay calm but regard a certain amount of anxiety as normal.

With regard to objective exam questions:
- Treat multiple choice questions as a series of T/F statements.
- Use the process of elimination with multiple choice questions. Eliminate distracters such as unfamiliar terms or phrases, jokes, extremely low or high numbers.
- Watch out for negative wording such as "not" and "unlikely" which may make a statement incorrect. (For example, if a statement says something is "not unlikely", this actually means "is likely" since two negatives equal a positive.)
- Be cautious about absolute wording. (For example, "always" and "never" are absolute words which tend to be in false statements whereas qualifying words such as "sometimes" and "seldom" tend to be in correct statements.)
- Remember all parts of a statement must be true for the statement to be true. Reasons which often begin with "because" or "since" can make a correct statement false because of the reason given.
- With multiple choice questions, there may be more than one correct answer so look for the best answer or "all of the above" answer.
- Watch out for changing answers unless you are certain.

With regard to essay exam questions:
- Identify key words that will determine how you answer the question. (For example, if the question asks you to "compare and contrast", you are being asked to tell how two things are alike *and* different.)
- Before you start writing, make a brief outline to ensure that your thoughts are organized and complete.
- Remember: Reasoning ability is just as important as factual accuracy when answering an essay question.

After the first examination in your Exercise Physiology class, if you did not perform as well as you would have liked, analyze the exam. Did most of the questions come from the text or the lectures? Where were your greatest sources of error (carelessness, lack of time, lack of understanding, uncertainty of directions, test anxiety)? How can you change your study strategies and test taking skills to perform better on the next exam? In addition to your Exercise Physiology instructor and teaching assistants, there are numerous resources available on your campus to help you with study skills in general (i.e. learning centers, study skills classes and counseling for test anxiety).

Hopefully the strategies included in this section and the following chapter-by-chapter learning objectives and sample exam questions will increase your enjoyment and success in Exercise Physiology.

Chapter 1: Physiology of Exercise in the U.S.

Chapter Learning Objectives

After studying this chapter you should be able to do the following:

1. Name the three Nobel Prize winners whose research work involved muscle or muscular exercise.
2. Describe the role of the Harvard Fatigue Laboratory in the history of exercise physiology in the United States.
3. Describe the factors influencing physical fitness in the United States over the past century.

Multiple Choice

Instructions: After reading the question, and all possible answers, select the letter of choice that *BEST* answers the question. *Read all possible answers because some questions may have more than one correct answer.* The correct answers are provided at the end of this chapter.

1. The three Nobel prize winners whose research work involved muscle or muscular exercise were
   a. A.V. Hill, August Krogh and Otto Meyerhof.
   b. J. S. Haldane, Christian Bohr and C. G. Douglas.
   c. D.B. Dill, L.J. Henderson and van Slyke.
   d. Steven Horvath, Sid Robinson and E. Asmussen.

2. The term "maximal oxygen uptake" was introduced in 1924 by
   a. Rudolpho Margaria.
   b. D. B. Dill.
   c. A.V. Hill.
   d. Otto Meyerhof.

3. Otto Meyerhof is recognized for his work on
   a. metabolism of citric acid.
   b. fat metabolism during long term work.
   c. metabolism of glucose.
   d. maximal oxygen uptake.

4. Which exercise physiology institute in Denmark bears the name of this Nobel prize winner?
   a. Rudolpho Margaria.
   b. August Krogh.
   c. A.V. Hill.
   d. Otto Meyerhof.

5. Two European scientists who did pioneering work in the role of O_2 and lactic acid in the control of breathing during exercise were
   a. Peter F. Scholander and Dr. Dudley Sargent.
   b. Steven Horvath and Thomas K. Cureton.
   c. C. G. Douglas and J. S. Haldane.
   d. Dr. Bruno Balke and T. H. Huxley.

6. The Harvard Fatigue Laboratory was open from
    a. 1927-1980.
    b. 1927-1947.
    c. 1947-1980.
    d. 1927-1937.

7. Dr. D. B. Dill's classic exercise physiology text is
    a. Life, Heat and Altitude.
    b. The Harvard Fatigue Laboratory.
    c. Maximal Oxygen Uptake.
    d. Physiology of Bodily Exercise.

8. A fellow of the Harvard Fatigue Laboratory who developed the chemical gas analyzer was
    a. Peter F. Scholander.
    b. Rudolpho Margaria.
    c. Dr. Bruno Balke.
    d. Otto Meyerhof.

9. President Kennedy expressed concerns about the nation's fitness in an article called
    a. Presidents Council on Physical Fitness.
    b. The soft American.
    c. AAHPERD's Physical Best.
    d. Corporate Fitness.

10. The Healthy People 2000 Health Objectives are concerned with
    a. increasing exercise.
    b. reducing dietary fat intake.
    c. decreasing tobacco use.
    d. All of the above.

11. In 1950 the number of Colleges or Universities that had research laboratories in departments of physical education was
    a. 151.
    b. 68.
    c. 58.
    d. 16.

12. Paralleling the interest in the physical fitness of America's youth in the 1960's was the rising concern about
    a. infectious disease.
    b. contagious disease.
    c. fitness testing.
    d. heart disease.

13. By 1969 how many Ph.D. students had completed their work under the direction of Thomas K. Cureton?
    a. 16.
    b. 68.
    c. 58.
    d. 30.

14. The acronym ACSM stands for
    a. The American College of Sports Medicine.
    b. The Association of Cardiovascular and Sports Medicine.
    c. The American Cardiovascular and Sports Meeting.
    d. The Association of Chemistry and Sports Medicine.

15. Which journal did the American Physiology Society publish in 1948 to bring together work in exercise and environmental physiology ?
    a. Journal of Biological Chemistry
    b. Medicine Science Sports and Exercise
    c. International Journal of Sports Medicine
    d. Journal of Applied Physiology

16. In 1969, ACSM first published the research journal
    a. Sports Medicine.
    b. Journal of Clinical Investigation.
    c. Medicine and Science in Sports and Exercise.
    d. Journal of Applied Physiology.

17. Three professional organizations that support the work of exercise physiology are
    a. American College of Sports Medicine, American Physiology Society, American Association of Health Physical Education and Recreation.
    b. American College of Sports Medicine, American Physiology Society, Medicine and Science in Sports.
    c. American Physiology Society, American Association of Health Physical Education and Recreation, Harvard Fatigue Laboratory.
    d. Medicine and Science in Sports, Journal of Applied Physiology, American College of Sports Medicine.

18. The term "basic research" usually refers to
    a. describing the responses of persons to exercise.
    b. describing the responses of persons to environmental factors.
    c. examining the mechanisms underlying a physiological issue.
    d. examining the responses of persons to nutritional factors.

19. The term "applied research" usually refers to
    a. describing the responses of persons to exercise.
    b. describing the responses of persons to environmental factors.
    c. describing the responses of persons to nutritional factors.
    d. All of the above.

20. Exercise physiology research is moving along a continuum to the domain of
    a. cell biology.
    b. epidemiology.
    c. whole body metabolism.
    d. role of exercise in disease prevention.

True and False

Instructions: Read each question carefully and determine if the statement is true or false. The correct answers to this exam are provided at the end of the chapter.

1. Christian Bohr is recognized for his work on the metabolism of glucose.

2. August Krogh received his Nobel Prize for his research on the function of the capillary circulation.

3. The canvas and rubber bag used to obtain ventilatory samples bears the name of J. S. Haldane.

4. The shift in the oxygen-hemoglobin dissociation curve due to the addition of CO_2 bears the name of Dr. Bruno Balke.

5. A focal point in the history of exercise physiology in the United States is the Harvard Fatigue Laboratory under the leadership of Dr. D. B. Dill.

6. In 1980 the public Health Service did not list physical fitness and exercise as one of 15 areas of concern related to improving the countries overall heath.

7. Concerns on the fitness of draftees during World War I and World War II failed to influence the type of physical education taught in schools.

8. Autopsies of soldiers killed during the Korean War did not show developed coronary artery disease.

9. In the 1950's Hans Kraus showed that American children out performed European children on a muscular fitness test.

10. President Kennedy expressed concern about the nation's fitness in a text entitled Health-Related Physical Fitness Test Manual.

11. The American Association for Health, Physical Education and Recreation (AAHPER) developed a youth fitness test in 1957.

12. In 1957 AAHPERD published a manual to distinguish performance testing from fitness testing.

13. The Healthy People 2000 Health Objectives recommend to reduce dietary fat intake to an average of 30% of calories or less.

14. In the last decade degenerative diseases have been shown to be related to poor health habits but are not responsible for more diseases than the classic infectious and contagious diseases.

15. Prior to the 1950's the two major societies concerned with the physiology of exercise were the American Physiological Society and the American Alliance for Health, Physical Education and Recreation.

16. Undergraduates should investigate graduate programs very carefully to make sure they meet their career goals.

17. Huxley once said " I often wish this phrase 'Applied Science' had never been invented".

18. AAHPER initiated certification programs in cardiac rehabilitation in 1975.

19. The Exercise Leader$_{sm}$ certification program is designed for fitness personnel who conduct exercise programs for the apparently healthy.

20. Graduate students are required to specialize earlier in their careers than in the past.

Answers

Multiple Choice
1. a
2. c
3. c
4. b
5. c
6. b
7. a
8. a
9. b
10. d
11. d
12. d
13. b
14. a
15. d
16. c
17. a
18. c
19. d
20. a

True and False
1. False
2. True
3. False
4. False
5. True
6. False
7. False
8. False
9. False
10. False
11. True
12. False
13. True
14. False
15. True
16. True
17. True
18. False
19. True
20. True

Chapter 2: Control of the Internal Environment

Chapter Learning Objectives

After studying this chapter you should be able to do the following:

1. Define the terms *homeostasis* and *steady state*.
2. Diagram and discuss a biological control system.
3. Give an example of a biological control system.
4. Explain the term *negative feedback*.
5. Define what is meant by the gain of a control system.

Multiple Choice

Instructions: After reading the question, and all possible answers, select the letter of choice that BEST answers the question. *Read all possible answers because some questions may have more than one correct answer.* The correct answers are provided at the end of this chapter.

1. During sixty minutes of submaximal exercise the body temperature reaches a plateau after 35-45 minutes, this is an example of
   a. homeostasis.
   b. effector center.
   c. steady state.
   d. changing internal environment.

2. Changes in arterial blood across time during resting conditions is an example of
   a. homeostasis.
   b. effector center.
   c. steady state.
   d. changing gain.

3. The overall goal of a control system is to regulate a physiological variable
   a. at or near a constant value.
   b. only in one system.
   c. at a changing value.
   d. only when exercising

4. The goal of "mechanistic" research is to
   a. determine why a specific control system operates.
   b. determine how a specific control system operates.
   c. determine when a specific control system operates.
   d. All of the above.

5. The general components of a biological control center are
   a. receptor, internal environment, effector.
   b. receptor, integrating center, input.
   c. input, stimulus, output.
   d. receptor, integrating center, effector.

6. Decreasing the original stimulus that triggered the control system is termed
   a. positive feedback.
   b. negative feedback.
   c. set point.
   d. gain.

7. The precision with which a control system maintains homeostasis is termed
   a. positive feedback.
   b. negative feedback.
   c. set point.
   d. gain.

8. The correction of disturbance and removal of stimulus is carried out by
   a. receptor.
   b. integrating center.
   c. effector.
   d. None of the above.

9. An example of the failure of a biological control system is
   a. insulin.
   b. blood glucose.
   c. steady state.
   d. None of the above.

10. The assessment of the response needed to correct a disturbance is made by the
    a. receptor.
    b. integrating center.
    c. effector.
    d. None of the above.

11. The amount of correction needed by a biological control system divided by the amount of abnormality that exists, is termed
    a. negative feedback.
    b. regulation.
    c. gain.
    d. steady state.

12. During heavy exercise or exercise in a hot or humid environment you may have
    a. disturbances in the internal environment.
    b. disruption of steady state.
    c. rapid responses of control systems.
    d. All of the above.

13. Severe disturbances in homeostasis result in fatigue and ultimately
    a. increase in performance.
    b. cessation of exercise.
    c. adjustment of gain.
    d. None of the above.

True and False

Instructions: Read each question carefully and determine if the statement is true or false. The correct answers to this exam are provided at the end of the chapter.

1. The term steady state is often applied to exercise when the physiological variable in question is changing.

2. Homeostasis represents a dynamic constancy.

3. The body has hundreds of different control systems.

4. Oscillation occurs in biological systems due to feedback.

7

5. Almost all organ systems of the body work to help maintain homeostasis.

6. The signal to begin the operation of a control system excites the integrating center.

7. A control system with a large gain is not able to correct alterations in homeostasis.

8. A high feedback gain in a control system means that it is more capable of maintaining homeostasis.

9. Most biological control systems operate in positive feedback.

10. An example of homeostatic control that uses negative feedback is the "baroreceptor system".

11. The control of blood glucose is an example of a positive feedback control system.

12. Muscular exercise is a test of the body's homeostatic control systems.

13. The body's control systems must respond slowly to prevent drastic alterations in the internal environment.

14. The body rarely maintains true homeostasis while performing intense or prolonged exercise in a hot humid environment.

Matching Terms and Definitions

Instructions: Consider each term carefully and select the correct definition below. The correct answers are provided at the end of the chapter.

Terms
1. biological control system
2. effector
3. gain
4. homeostasis
5. integrating center
6. negative feedback
7. receptor
8. steady state

Definitions
a. Responsible for processing the information from the receptors and then issues an appropriate response relative to it's set point.
b. The amount of correction that a control system is capable of achieving.
c. A control system capable of maintaining homeostasis within a cell or organ system in a living creature.
d. The response from a control system that reduces the size of the stimulus.
e. Maintenance of a constant internal environment.
f. A specialized portion of an afferent neuron that is sensitive to a form of energy in the environment.
g. A relatively constant internal environment, may not represent homeostasis.
h. Organ or body tissue that responds to stimulation by an integrating center.

Answers

Multiple Choice

1. c
2. a
3. a
4. b
5. d
6. b
7. d
8. c
9. d
10. b
11. c
12. d
13. b

True and False

1. False
2. True
3. True
4. True
5. True
6. False
7. False
8. True
9. False
10. True
11. False
12. True
13. False
14. True

Terms and Definitions

1. c
2. h
3. b
4. e
5. a
6. d
7. f
8. g

Chapter 3: Bioenergetics

Chapter Learning Objectives

After studying this chapter, you should be able to do the following:

1. Discuss the function of the cell membrane, nucleus and mitochondria.
2. Define the following terms: 1) endergonic reactions, 2) exergonic reactions, 3) coupled reactions, and 4) bioenergetics.
3. Describe the role of enzymes as catalysts in cellular chemical reactions.
4. List and discuss the nutrients that are used as fuels during exercise.
5. Identify the high energy phosphates.
6. Discuss the biochemical pathways involved in anaerobic ATP production.
7. Discuss the aerobic production of ATP.
8. Describe the general scheme used to regulate metabolic pathways involved in bioenergetics.
9. Discuss the interaction between aerobic and anaerobic ATP production during exercise.
10. Identify the enzymes that are considered rate limiting in glycolysis and the Krebs cycle.

Multiple Choice

Instructions: After reading the question, and all possible answers, select the letter of choice that *BEST* answers the question. *Read all possible answers because some questions may have more than one correct answer.* The correct answers are provided at the end of this chapter.

1. In order to continue to contract, muscle cells must have
   a. carbohydrates.
   b. oxygen.
   c. ATP .
   d. All of the above.

2. The synthesis of molecules is called
   a. catabolism.
   b. metabolism.
   c. anabolism.
   d. All of the above.

3. Protein synthesis within the cell is regulated by
   a. cytoplasm.
   b. organelles.
   c. genes.
   d. cell membrane.

4. The speed of chemical reactions that occur within the body are regulated by
   a. exergonic reactions.
   b. endergonic reactions.
   c. entropy.
   d. enzymes.

5. Increasing the rate of chemical reactions is achieved by _____ the energy of activation.
   a. changing
   b. lowering
   c. raising
   d. not altering

6. The ability of an enzyme to bind to a particular substrate is achieved by
   a. active sites.
   b. reactant molecules.
   c. a catalyst.
   d. a key.

7. During exercise, the primary nutrients used for energy are
   a. fats.
   b. carbohydrates.
   c. proteins.
   d. Both a and b are correct

8. An example of a carbohydrate that is both found in the diet and released from the liver is
   a. sucrose.
   b. fructose.
   c. glucose.
   d. maltose.

9. What duration of continuous exercise might deplete total muscle glycogen stores
   a. few hours.
   b. few days.
   c. few minutes.
   d. few seconds.

10. How much energy does one gram of fat contain
    a. 4 kcal.
    b. 18 kcal.
    c. 12 kcal.
    d. 9 kcal.

11. In order for proteins to be used as substrates they must first be broken down
    a. by glucose.
    b. by glycogen.
    c. to amino acids.
    d. to peptide bonds.

12. The immediate source of energy for muscular contraction is
    a. adenosine triphosphate.
    b. adenosine monophosphate.
    c. adenosine diphosphate.
    d. inorganic phosphate.

13. The enzyme responsible for the breaking of ATP into energy and inorganic phosphate is
    a. ATPase.
    b. ATP.
    c. lactate dehydrogenase.
    d. creatine phosphate.

14. Muscle cells can produce ATP by
    a. creatine phosphate pathway.
    b. glycolysis.
    c. aerobic metabolism.
    d. All of the above

15. Glycolysis produces a net gain of how many ATP molecules per glucose molecules ?
    a. one
    b. two
    c. three
    d. four

16. The purpose of the energy investment phase of glycolysis is
    a. to phosphorylate inorganic phosphate.
    b. to phosphorylate substrates using ATP.
    c. to store ATP.
    d. to form glycogen.

17. NAD is reformed from NADH by
    a. shuttling of hydrogens from NADH into the mitochondria.
    b. pyruvic acid can accept hydrogens to form lactic acid.
    c. shuttling of O_2 into the mitochondria.
    d. Both a and b are correct.

18. The chemiosmotic hypothesis describes how
    a. ATP is produced aerobically.
    b. ATP is formed via hydrogen ion diffusion.
    c. hydrogen ions are pumped across the inner mitochondrial membrane.
    d. All of the above.

19. The primary function of the Krebs cycle is to
    a. produce ATP.
    b. complete the oxidation of carbohydrates, fats and proteins.
    c. prepare acetyl-CoA.
    d. All of the above.

20. The two anaerobic metabolic pathways are
    a. Krebs cycle and the electron transport chain.
    b. Krebs cycle and the ATP-PC system.
    c. ATP-PC system and the electron transport chain.
    d. ATP-PC system and glycolysis.

21. The majority of electrons that enter the electron transport chain come from
    a. NADH and FADH formed in the Krebs cycle.
    b. degradation of glucose via glycolysis.
    c. resynthesis of ATP from ADP and Pi.
    d. combination of oxygen and hydrogen.

22. The aerobic metabolism of one molecule of glucose results in the production of
    a. 38 ATP.
    b. 39 ATP.
    c. 8 ATP.
    d. 16 ATP.

23. Phosphocreatine breakdown is regulated by
    a. creatine kinase.
    b. phosphofructokinase.
    c. isocitrate dehydrogenase.
    d. None of the above.

24. Important regulatory enzymes in carbohydrate metabolism are
    a. creatine kinase and phosphofructokinase.
    b. phosphofructokinase and phosphorylase.
    c. isocitrate dehydrogenase and phosphofructokinase.
    d. creatine kinase and phosphorylase.

25. Metabolic pathways that produce ATP are generally regulated by levels of
    a. ADP.
    b. ATP.
    c. cytochrome oxidase.
    d. Both a and b are correct.

True and False

Instructions: Read each question carefully and determine if the statement is true or false. The correct answers to this exam are provided at the end of the chapter.

1. All cells possess the ability to convert foodstuffs into a biologically usable form of energy.

2. All the chemical reactions that occur throughout the body are collectively called catabolism.

3. Energy transfer in the body occurs via the releasing of energy trapped within chemical bonds.

4. Enzymes increase the rate of product formation.

5. Protein contributes only a small amount to the total energy during exercise.

6. Glycogen is a disaccharide that is formed by combining two monosaccharides.

7. Glycogen is stored only in the liver.

8. Glycogen synthesis is an ongoing process within cells.

9. During exercise, individual muscle cells break down glycogen to glucose.

10. The entire triglyceride molecule is a useful source of energy for the body.

11. The formation of adenosine triphosphate occurs by combining adenosine monophosphate and inorganic phosphate.

12. Muscles store large amounts of ATP.

13. The simplest and most rapid method of producing ATP is via aerobic metabolism.

14. Muscle cells can produce ATP by any one of two metabolic pathways.

15. The ATP-PC system provides energy for muscular contraction at the onset of exercise.

16. Hydrogen carriers transport energy for generation of ATP in the mitochondria.

17. The reason for lactic acid formation is the recycling of NAD.

18. The anaerobic breakdown of glycogen yields two ATP.

13

19. Beta oxidation is the process of oxidizing fatty acids to form glucose.

20. The efficiency of aerobic respiration is around 40%.

21. The rate limiting enzyme of the Krebs cycle is cytochrome oxidase.

22. The end result of the electron transport chain is the formation of NADH and FADH.

23. Approximately 90% of the energy to perform a 100-meter dash would come from anaerobic systems.

24. The shorter the activity the greater the contribution of anaerobic energy production.

25. The most important rate limiting enzyme in glycolysis is isocitrate dehydrogenase.

Matching Terms and Definitions

Instructions: Consider each term carefully and select the correct definition below. The correct answers are provided at the end of the chapter.

Terms and Definitions (Group 1)

Terms (Group 1)
1. adenosine diphosphate (ADP)
2. adenosine triphosphate (ATP)
3. aerobic
4. anaerobic
5. ATPase
6. ATP-PC system
7. beta oxidation
8. bioenergetics
9. cell membrane
10. chemiosmotic hypothesis
11. coupled reactions
12. cytoplasm
13. electron transport chain
14. endergonic reactions
15. energy of activation
16. enzymes
17. exergonic reactions

Definitions (Group 1)
a. Breakdown of free fatty acids to form acetyl-CoA.
b. The metabolic pathway involving muscle stores of ATP and the use of creatine phosphate to rephosphorylate ATP.
c. A series of cytochromes in the mitochondria that are responsible for oxidative phosphorylation.
d. Energy required to initiate a chemical reaction.
e. A molecule that combines with inorganic phosphate to form ATP.
f. The contents of the cell surrounding the nucleus.
g. Chemical reactions that release energy.
h. The high energy phosphate compound synthesized and used by cells to release energy for cellular work.
i. Chemical processes involved in the production of ATP.
j. Without oxygen.
k. The lipid-bilayer envelope that encloses cells.
l. Proteins that lower the energy of activation and therefore catalyze chemical reactions.
m. In the presence of oxygen.
n. The linking of energy-liberating chemical reactions to drive energy-requiring reactions.
o. Enzyme capable of breaking down ATP to form ADP + Pi + energy.
p. Energy-requiring reactions.
q. The mechanism to explain the aerobic formation of ATP in mitochondria.

Terms and Definitions (Group 2)

Terms (Group 2)
1. FAD
2. glucose
3. glycogen
4. glycogenolysis
5. glycolysis
6. inorganic
7. inorganic phosphate (P_i)
8. isocitrate dehydrogenase
9. Krebs cycle
10. lactic acid
11. mitochondrion
12. molecular biology
13. NAD
14. nucleus
15. organic
16. oxidative phosphorylation
17. phosphocreatine (PC)
18. phosphofructokinase

Definitions (Group 2)
a. Rate-limiting enzyme in the Krebs cycle that is inhibited by ATP and stimulated by ADP and Pi.
b. A metabolic pathway in the cytoplasm of the cell that results in the degradation of glucose into pyruvate or lactate.
c. Mitochondrial process in which inorganic phosphate is coupled to ADP.
d. Rate limiting enzyme in glycolysis.
e. The membrane bound organelle that contains most of the cell's DNA.
f. Serves as an electron carrier in bioenergetics.
g. Relating to substances that do not contain carbon.
h. Metabolic pathway in the mitochondria in which energy is transferred for subsequent production of ATP in the electron transport chain.
i. A simple sugar that is transported via the blood and metabolized by tissues.
j. A stimulator of cellular metabolism; split off, along with ADP from ATP when energy is released.
k. The subcellular organelle responsible for the production of ATP with oxygen.
l. Coenzyme that transfers hydrogen and the energy associated with those hydrogens.
m. A glucose polymer synthesized in cells as a means of storing carbohydrate.
n. Describes substances that contain carbon.
o. Branch of biochemistry involved with the study of gene structure and function.
p. The breakdown of glycogen into glucose.
q. An end product of glucose metabolism in the glycolytic pathway; formed in conditions of inadequate oxygen.
r. Compound that resynthesizes ATP from ADP

Answers

Multiple Choice
1. c
2. c
3. c
4. d
5. b
6. a
7. d
8. c
9. a
10. d
11. c
12. a
13. a
14. d
15. b
16. b
17. d
18. d
19. b
20. d
21. a
22. a
23. a
24. b
25. d

True and False

1. True
2. False
3. True
4. True
5. True
6. False
7. False
8. True
9. True
10. True
11. False
12. False
13. False
14. False
15. True
16. True
17. True
18. False
19. False
20. True
21. False
22. False
23. True
24. True
25. False

Terms and Definitions (Group 1)

1. e
2. h
3. m
4. j
5. o
6. b
7. a
8. i
9. k
10. q
11. n
12. f
13. c
14. p
15. d
16. l
17. g

Terms and Definitions (Group 2)

1. f
2. i
3. m
4. p
5. b
6. g
7. j
8. a
9. h
10. q
11. k
12. o
13. l
14. e
15. n
16. c
17. r
18. d

Chapter 4: Exercise Metabolism

Chapter Learning Objectives

After studying this chapter you should be able to do the following:

1. Discuss the relationship between exercise intensity/duration and the bioenergetic pathways that are most responsible for production of ATP during various types of exercise.
2. Define the term oxygen deficit.
3. Define the term lactate threshold.
4. Discuss several possible explanations for the sudden rise in blood-lactate concentration during incremental exercise.
5. List the factors that regulate fuel selection during different types of exercise.
6. Explain why fat metabolism is dependent on carbohydrate metabolism.
7. Define the term oxygen debt.
8. Give the physiological explanation for the observation that the O_2 debt is greater following intense exercise when compared to the O_2 debt following light exercise.

Multiple Choice

Instructions: After reading the question, and all possible answers, select the letter of choice that *BEST* answers the question. *Read all possible answers because some questions may have more than one correct answer.* The correct answers are provided at the end of this chapter.

1. During heavy exercise the body's total energy expenditure may increase by
   a. twice that at rest.
   b. fifteen to twenty five times that at rest.
   c. two hundred times that at rest.
   d. None of the above.

2. Trained individuals have a lower oxygen deficit, this may be due to
   a. having a lower VO_2 max.
   b. having a greater reliance on anaerobic pathways.
   c. the involvement of more energy systems.
   d. having a better developed aerobic bioenergetic capacity.

3. Which of the following groups of activities use energy derived predominantly from the ATP-PC system?
   a. golf swing, tennis serve, 400m swim.
   b. 400m sprint, 50m swim, triple jump.
   c. gymnastics vault, softball pitch, high jump.
   d. 1500m swim, 5000m run, 90 min. soccer match.

4. The drift upward of VO_2 during steady state exercise is primarily due to
   a. rising blood levels of hormones.
   b. decreasing blood levels of hormones.
   c. increasing body temperature.
   d. decreasing body temperature.

5. The physiological factors that influence VO_2 max are
   a. the delivery of oxygen to the muscle.
   b. the uptake of oxygen by the muscle.
   c. genetics and exercise training.
   d. All of the above.

6. A factor that contributes to excess post exercise oxygen consumption is
   a. decreased body temperature.
   b. resynthesis of creatine phosphate in muscle.
   c. glycolysis.
   d. None of the above.

7. The lactate threshold in untrained subjects appears at around
   a. 50-60% VO_2max.
   b. 65-80% VO_2max.
   c. 40-50% VO_2max.
   d. 80-90% VO_2max.

8. A rise in blood lactic acid concentration can occur due to
   a. excess O_2 available in the mitochondria.
   b. increase in lactic acid production.
   c. decrease in lactic acid removal.
   d. Both b and c are correct.

9. A noninvasive technique that is commonly used to estimate substrate contribution to ATP production is by measuring
   a. VO_2 max.
   b. respiratory exchange ratio.
   c. lactate threshold.
   d. anaerobic threshold.

10. During low intensity exercise (i.e., <30% VO_2 max) the primary fuel source for muscle is
    a. proteins.
    b. carbohydrates.
    c. fats.
    d. glucose.

11. To measure fuel utilization during exercise it is necessary to have the subject
    a. exercise at steady state.
    b. exercise at maximal intensity.
    c. exercise at the lactate threshold.
    d. exercise at the anaerobic threshold.

12. As exercise increases in intensity there is a shift from fat to _____ metabolism.
    a. protein
    b. carbohydrate
    c. glycerol
    d. aerobic

13 The shift from fat to carbohydrate metabolism is regulated by
   a. type of fiber recruited.
   b. level of epinephrine.
   c. the size and number of mitochondria.
   d. Both a and b are correct.

14. The primary determinant of the substrate used during exercise is
    a. the type of muscle cell.
    b. the availability of the fuel.
    c. hormone levels.
    d. None of the above.

15. Most of the carbohydrate used as a substrate during exercise comes from
    a. liver glycogen.
    b. muscle glycogen.
    c. fat oxidation.
    d. blood glucose.

16. During the first hour of submaximal prolonged exercise, most of the carbohydrate metabolized comes from
    a. liver glycogen.
    b. muscle glycogen.
    c. fat oxidation.
    d. blood glucose.

17. The mobilization of free fatty acids into the blood is inhibited by
    a. insulin.
    b. glycogen.
    c. lactic acid.
    d. Both a and c are correct

18. What duration of exercise is generally required to significantly deplete muscle glycogen stores?
    a. 120 min.
    b. 240 min.
    c. 10 min.
    d. 2 min.

19. Fatigue results after depletion of carbohydrate stores due to the reduction
    a. in the muscle concentration of pyruvic acid.
    b. of Krebs cycle intermediates.
    c. of Krebs cycle activity.
    d. All of the above.

20. The portion of the oxygen debt that is responsible for the conversion of lactic acid to glycogen is around
    a. 10%.
    b. 20%.
    c. 30% .
    d. 40%.

True and False

Instructions: Read each question carefully and determine if the statement is true or false. The correct answers to this exam are provided at the end of the chapter.

1. In the transition from rest to moderate exercise, oxygen consumption reaches a steady state within 30 seconds.

2. VO_2 max is not a valid measure of cardiovascular fitness.

3. Oxygen uptake increases as a linear function of the work rate until VO_2 max is reached.

4. The formation of lactic acid can occur in the presence of sufficient oxygen.

5. Lactic acid can be converted back to pyruvic acid under appropriate conditions.

6. The LDH isozyme found in slow-twitch fibers has a greater affinity for attaching to pyruvic acid.

7. The lactate threshold can not be used as a predictor of success in distance running.

8. Proteins contribute less than 2% of the fuel used during exercise of less than one hour.

9. During prolonged exercise, after 30 minutes there is a gradual shift from fat to carbohydrate metabolism.

10. During high intensity short term exercise (i.e., 2 to 20 seconds), the muscles ATP production is dominated by the ATP-PC system.

11. During prolonged exercise (i.e., 3 to 5 hours) the total contribution of protein to the fuel supply may reach 5% - 50%.

12. Fats are used as the primary fuel during high intensity exercise.

13. Lactate can be produced in one tissue and then transported to another.

14. Epinephrine promotes carbohydrate metabolism.

15. Free fatty acids can directly enter the Krebs cycle.

16. Exercise above the lactate threshold results in a reduction in blood levels of free fatty acids available as a substrate.

17. When carbohydrate stores are depleted in muscle, the rate at which fat is metabolized is decreased.

18. Oxygen uptake is greater, and remains elevated for a longer time period following high intensity exercise than low intensity exercise.

19. The cycle of lactate to glucose occurs between the muscle and the kidney.

20. At the beginning of exercise the contribution of plasma FFA and muscle triglycerides is equal.

Matching Terms and Definitions

Instructions: Consider each term carefully and select the correct definition below. The correct answers are provided at the end of the chapter.

Terms
1. anaerobic threshold
2. Cori cycle
3. EPOC
4. free fatty acid
5. gluconeogenesis
6. graded or incremental exercise test
7. lactate threshold
8. lipase
9. lipolysis
10. maximal oxygen uptake (VO_2 max)
11. oxygen debt
12. oxygen deficit
13. respiratory exchange ratio (R)

Definitions
a. Related to the replacement of creatine phosphate, lactic acid related to synthesis to glucose and elevated body temperature, catecholamines and heart rate.
b. A type of fat that combines with glycerol to form triglycerides.
c. The breakdown of triglycerides in adipose tissue to free fatty acids and glycerol.
d. An enzyme responsible for the breakdown of triglycerides.
e. The level of oxygen consumption at which there is a rapid and systematic increase in blood lactate concentration.
f. The greatest rate of oxygen uptake by the body.
g. The lag in oxygen uptake at the beginning of exercise.
h. Often referred to as oxygen debt.
i. A point during a graded exercise test when the blood lactate concentration increases abruptly.
j. An exercise test involving a progessive increase in work rate over time.
k. The ratio of carbon dioxide to oxygen production.
l. Synthesis of glucose from amino acids, lactate, glycerol, and other short chain carbon molecules.
m. The cycle of lactate to glucose between the muscle and the liver.

Answers

Multiple Choice
1. b
2. d
3. c
4. c
5. d
6. b
7. a
8. d
9. b
10. c
11. a
12. b
13. d
14. b
15. b
16. b
17. d
18. a
19. b
20. d

True and False
1. False
2. False
3. True
4. True
5. True
6. False
7. False
8. True
9. True
10. True
11. False
12. False
13. True
14. True
15. True
16. True
17. True
18. True
19. False
20. True

Terms and Definitions

1. e or i
2. m
3. h
4. b
5. l
6. j
7. i or e
8. d
9. c
10. f
11. a
12. g
13. k

Chapter 5: Hormonal Responses to Exercise

Chapter Learning Objectives

After studying this chapter you should be able to do the following:

1. Describe the concept of hormone-receptor interaction.
2. Identify the four factors influencing the concentration of a hormone in the blood.
3. Describe the mechanism by which steroid hormones act on cells.
4. Describe the "second messenger" hypothesis of hormone action.
5. Describe the role of the hypothalamus-releasing factors in the control of hormone secretion from the anterior pituitary.
6. Describe the relationship of the hypothalamus to the secretion of hormones from the posterior pituitary gland.
7. Identify the site of release, stimulus for release, and the predominant action of the following hormones: epinephrine, norepinephrine, glucagon, insulin, cortisol, aldosterone, thyroxine, growth hormone, estrogen and testosterone.
8. Discuss the use of testosterone (an anabolic steroid) and growth hormone on muscle growth and their potential side effects.
9. Contrast the role of plasma catecholamines with intracellular factors in the mobilization of muscle glycogen during exercise.
10. Graphically describe the changes in the following hormones during graded and prolonged exercise and discuss how those changes influence the four mechanisms used to maintain the blood glucose concentration: insulin, glucagon, cortisol, growth hormone, epinephrine, and norepinephrine.
11. Describe the effect of changing hormone and substrate levels in the blood on the mobilization of free fatty acids from adipose tissue.

Multiple Choice

Instructions: After reading the question, and all possible answers, select the letter of choice that *BEST* answers the question. *Read all possible answers because some questions may have more than one correct answer.* The correct answers are provided at the end of this chapter.

1. The two major systems involved in the control of homeostatic bodily functions are the
   a. endocrine and nervous systems.
   b. endocrine and cardiovascular systems.
   c. endocrine and renal systems.
   d. endocrine and metabolic systems.

2. The effect a hormone exerts on a tissue is directly related to
   a. the chemical structure of the hormone.
   b. concentration of the hormone in the plasma.
   c. number of receptors available.
   d. Both b and c are correct.

3. The magnitude of the effect a hormone has is directly related to
   a. the plasma volume.
   b. the rate of hormone secretion .
   c. plasma hormone concentration.
   d. All of the above.

4. If a hormone-receptor interaction activates a Ca^{++} ion channel and Ca^{++} enters the cell it will often bind to
   a. phosphodiesterase.
   b. calmodulin.
   c. cyclic AMP.
   d. 5'AMP.

5. Examples of second messengers in the events following a hormones binding to a receptor are
   a. cyclic GAMP, caffeine.
   b. epinephrine, inositol triphosphate.
   c. diacyclglycerol, phospholipase C.
   d. cyclic AMP, Ca^{++}-calmodulin.

6. When G protein activates adenylate cyclase what molecule is formed from ATP?
   a. phosphodiesterase.
   b. cyclic AMP.
   c. calmodulin.
   d. calcium.

7. Hormones released from the anterior pituitary include
   a. growth hormone, anti diuretic hormone.
   b. thyroid stimulating hormone, thyroxine.
   c. prolactin, adrenocorticotropic hormone.
   d. luteinizing hormone, somatomedins.

8. Catecholamines are secreted from the
   a. adrenal cortex.
   b. adrenal medulla.
   c. parathyroid gland.
   d. None of the above.

9. Aldosterone is secreted by the
   a. adrenal cortex.
   b. adrenal medulla.
   c. parathyroid gland.
   d. none of the above.

10. At what approximate exercise intensity does increases in blood levels of aldosterone, renin and angiotensin II occur?
    a. 20%.
    b. 30%.
    c. 50%.
    d. 70%.

11. High blood levels of glucocorticoids can result in
    a. muscle atrophy.
    b. muscle hyperplasia.
    c. muscle hypertrophy.
    d. muscle hypoplasia.

12. The initial event at the onset of exercise activating phosphorylase activity is
    a. increased intracellular cAMP.
    b. increased intracellular calcium.
    c. increased release of epinephrine.
    d. None of the above.

13. Chronic exercise training _____ testosterone levels in males.
   a. increases
   b. decreases
   c. decreases then increases
   d. does not effect

14. The maintenance of plasma glucose during exercise can be accomplished by
   a. liver glycogenolysis.
   b. mobilization of FFA.
   c. liver gluconeogenesis.
   d. All of the above.

15. Examples of slow acting hormones responsible for the maintenance of plasma glucose are
   a. epinephrine and norepinephrine.
   b. insulin and glucagon.
   c. cortisol and growth hormone.
   d. none of the above.

16. The increased uptake of glucose when insulin decreases is due to
   a. decreasing intracellular calcium.
   b. increased membrane permeability.
   c. increased number of glucose transporters.
   d. decreasing catecholamines.

17. Epinephrine acts to maintain blood glucose by binding to
   a. alpha receptors on the liver.
   b. alpha cells of the pancreas.
   c. beta receptors on the liver.
   d. beta cells of the pancreas.

18. How does exercise alter the rate of glucose transport into muscle ?
   a. through high intramuscular Ca^{++}
   b. through decreasing glucagon levels
   c. through increasing insulin levels
   d. None of the above

19. An effect of endurance training that results in sparing carbohydrate stores is
   a. decreasing epinephrine concentration.
   b. decreasing lactate concentration.
   c. decreasing insulin concentration .
   d. decreasing glucagon concentration.

20. Decreasing plasma FFA concentration during heavy exercise is due to
   a. high levels of lactate.
   b. increased blood flow to adipose tissue.
   c. increased albumin .
   d. All of the above.

True and False

Instructions: Read each question carefully and determine if the statement is true or false. The correct answers to this exam are provided at the end of the chapter.

1. Most endocrine glands are under the control of more than one type of input.

2. Each specific receptor can recognize more than one hormone.

3. Steroid hormones are unable to diffuse through cell membranes.

4. Cyclic AMP is inactivated by phosphodiesterase.

5. Growth hormone is released from the posterior pituitary and is essential for normal growth.

6. The release of hormones from the anterior pituitary is controlled by neural signals.

7. Chronic use of growth hormone has been shown to lead to a shortened life span.

8. Parathyroid hormone is the primary hormone responsible for plasma Ca^{++} regulation.

9. Thyroid hormones are important for maintaining the metabolic rate.

10. Testosterone can promote protein synthesis.

11. There are different plasma concentrations of estrogen during exercise depending on the menstrual cycle stage.

12. Thyroxine levels change dramatically when a person starts exercising.

13. Norepinephrine is the adrenal medulla's primary secretion.

14. Cortisol secretion increases as exercise intensity increases.

15. Plasma insulin increases with increasing duration of exercise.

16. Catecholamines work via second messengers.

17. Plasma glucagon has a greater increase in trained individuals with increasing duration of exercise.

18. The ability of exercising muscle to take up glucose is dependent on insulin.

19. Glucagon promotes the storage of glucose.

20. Lactic acid inhibits the mobilization of free fatty acids.

Matching Terms and Definitions

Instructions: Consider each term carefully and select the correct definition below. The correct answers are provided at the end of the chapter.

Matching Terms and Definitions (Group 1)

Terms (Group 1)
1. acromegaly
2. adenylate cyclase
3. adrenal cortex
4. adrenocorticotropic hormone (ACTH)
5. aldosterone
6. alpha receptors
7. anabolic steroid
8. androgenic steroid
9. androgens
10. angiotensin I and II
11. anterior pituitary
12. antidiuretic hormone (ADH)
13. beta receptors
14. calcitonin
15. calmodulin
16. catecholamines
17. cortisol
18. cyclic AMP
19. diabetes mellitus

Definitions (Group 1)
a. Male sex hormones synthesized in the testes.
b. Enzyme found in cell membranes that catalyzes the conversion of ATP to cyclic AMP.
c. Polypeptides formed by the action of renin and a converting enzyme in the lung.
d. Subtype of adrenergic receptors located on cell membranes of selected tissues.
e. Caused by oversecretion of growth hormone.
f. Condition characterized by high blood glucose levels due to inadequate insulin.
g. Part of second messenger system involving calcium that results in changes in the activity of intracellular enzymes.
h. Glucocorticoid released from the adrenal cortex upon stimulation by ACTH.
i. Adrenergic receptor that combines mainly with epinephrine.
j. Compound that has the qualities of an androgen.
k. Substance produced from ATP through the action of adenylate cyclase that alters several chemical processes within the cell.
l. Synthesizes and secretes corticosteroid hormones.
m. Organic compounds that include epinephrine, norepinephrine and dopamine.
n. Prescription drug that has an anabolic or growth stimulating effect.
o. Secreted by the anterior pituitary gland and stimulates the adrenal cortex.
p. Hormone released by the thyroid gland that plays a minor role in calcium metabolism.
q. Corticosteroid hormone involved in the regulation of electrolyte balance.
r. Hormone secreted by the posterior pituitary that promotes water retention by the kidney.
s. Secretes FSH, LH, ACTH, TSH, GH and prolactin.

Terms and Definitions (Group 2)

Terms (Group 2)
1. diacyclglycerol
2. endocrine gland
3. endorphin
4. epinephrine (E)
5. estrogens
6. follicle-stimulating hormone (FSH)
7. G protein
8. glucagon
9. glucocorticoids
10. growth hormone (GH)
11. hormone
12. hypothalamic somatostatin
13. hypothalamus
14. inositol triphosphate
15. insulin
16. luteinizing hormone (LH)
17. mineralcorticoids
18. neuroendocrinology
19. norepinephrine (NE)
20. pancreas

Definitions (Group 2)

a. Study of the role of the nervous and endocrine systems in the automatic regulation of the internal environment.

b. Female sex hormones including estradiole and estrone.

c. Hormone that stimulates ovulation in the middle of the menstrual cycle.

d. Molecule derived from a membrane bound phospholipid that activates protein kinase C and alters cellular activity.

e. Chemical substance that is synthesized and released by an endocrine gland and transported to a target organ via the blood.

f. Any one of a group of hormones produced by the adrenal cortex that influences carbohydrate, fat and protein metabolism.

g. Hormone synthesized by the adrenal medulla, also called adrenaline.

h. Hormone synthesized and secreted by the anterior pituitary gland that stimulates the growth of the skeleton and soft tissues during the growing years.

i. Gland that produces and secretes its products directly into the blood or interstitial fluid.

j. Hormone and neurotransmitter released from postganglionic nerve endings and the adrenal medulla.

k. Neuropeptide produced by the pituitary gland having pain suppressing activity.

l. Hormone that inhibits growth hormone secretion.

m. Steroid hormones released from the adrenal cortex that are responsible for Na^+ and K^+ regulation.

n. Molecule derived from a membrane bound phospholipid that causes calcium release from intracellular stores and alters cellular activity.

o. Hormone secreted by the anterior pituitary gland that stimulates the development of an ovarian follicle in the female and sperm in the male.

p. Hormone produced by the pancreas that acts to increase blood glucose and free fatty acid levels.

q. Hormone released from the beta cells of the islets of Langerhans in response to elevated blood glucose.

r. Brain structure that integrates many physiological functions to maintain homeostasis.

s. Gland that contains both exocrine and endocrine portions.

t. Link between the hormone-receptor interaction on the membranes surface and the subsequent events inside the cell.

Terms and Definitions (Group 3)

Terms (Group 3)

1. phosphodiesterase
2. phospholipase C
3. pituitary gland
4. posterior pituitary gland
5. prolactin
6. protein kinase C
7. releasing hormone
8. renin
9. second messenger
10. sex steroids
11. somatomedins
12. somatostatin
13. steroids
14. testosterone
15. thyroid gland
16. thyroid stimulating hormone (TSH)
17. thyroxine (T_4)
18. triiodothyronine (T_3)

Definitions (Group 3)

a. Steroid hormone produced in the testes involved in growth and development of reproductive tissues, sperm and secondary sex characteristics.

b. Hormone secreted from the anterior pituitary that increases milk production from the breast.

c. Enzyme that catalyzes the breakdown of cyclic AMP.

d. Hormone secreted from the thyroid gland containing four iodine atoms which stimulates the metabolic rate.
e. Hormone produced in the hypothalamus that inhibits growth hormone release.
f. Hypothalamic hormones released from neurons into the anterior pituitary that control the release of hormones from that gland.
g. Membrane bound enzyme that hydrolyzes phosphotidylinositol into inositol triphosphate.
h. A molecule or ion that increases in a cell as a result of an interaction between a first messenger and a receptor.
i. Part of second messenger system that is activated by diacyclglycerol and results in the activation of proteins in the cell.
j. Class of lipids that include the hormones testosterone and cortisol.
k. Endocrine gland located in the neck that secretes T_3 and T_4.
l. Hormone secreted from the thyroid gland containing three iodine atoms which stimulates the metabolic rate.
m. Gland at the base of the hypothalamus.
n. Hormone released from the anterior pituitary gland which stimulates the thyroid gland to increase it's secretion of T_3 and T_4.
o. Group of hormones, androgens and estrogens, secreted by the adrenal cortex and the gonads.
p. Group of growth-stimulating peptides released primarily from the liver in response to growth hormone.
q. Enzyme secreted by special cells in the kidney that converts renin substrate to angiotensin I.
r. Secretes oxytocin and ADH that are produced in the hypothalamus.

Answers

Multiple Choice

1. a
2. d
3. d
4. b
5. d
6. b
7. c
8. b
9. a
10. c
11. a
12. b
13. b
14. d
15. b
16. c
17. c
18. a
19. b
20. a

True and False

1. True
2. False
3. False
4. True
5. False
6. False
7. True
8. True
9. True
10. True
11. True
12. False
13. False
14. True
15. False
16. True
17. False
18. False
19. False
20. True

Terms and Definitions (Group 1)	Terms and Definitions (Group 2)	Terms and Definitions (Group 3)
1. e	1. d	1. c
2. b	2. i	2. g
3. l	3. k	3. m
4. o	4. g	4. r
5. q	5. b	5. b
6. d	6. o	6. i
7. n	7. t	7. f
8. j	8. p	8. q
9. a	9. f	9. h
10. c	10. h	10. o
11. s	11. e	11. p
12. r	12. l	12. e
13. i	13. r	13. j
14. p	14. n	14. a
15. g	15. q	15. k
16. m	16. c	16. n
17. h	17. m	17. d
18. k	18. a	18. l
19. f	19. j	
	20. s	

Chapter 6: Measurement of Work, Power and Energy Expenditure

Chapter Learning Objectives

After studying this chapter you should be able to do the following:

1. Define the terms *work, power, energy,* and *net efficiency.*
2. Give a brief explanation of the procedure used to calculate work performed during: a) cycle ergometer exercise and b) treadmill exercise.
3. Describe the concept behind the measurement of energy expenditure using: a) direct calorimetry and b) indirect calorimetry.
4. Discuss the procedure to estimate energy expenditure during horizontal treadmill walking and running.
5. Define the following terms: a) *kilogram-meter,* b) *relative VO$_2$,* c) *MET,* and d) *open-circuit spirometry.*
6. Describe the procedure used to calculate net efficiency during steady state exercise.

Multiple Choice

Instructions: After reading the question, and all possible answers, select the letter of choice that *BEST* answers the question. *Read all possible answers because some questions may have more than one correct answer.* The correct answers are provided at the end of this chapter.

1. The SI system of quantifying units is used because
   a. it ensures standardization.
   b. makes comparisons of published data easier.
   c. it has been endorsed by numerous journals.
   d. All of the above.

2. The units used for work are
   a. Newtons or Newton-meters.
   b. joules or kilo pond-meters.
   c. watts or joules.
   d. Newton-meters or kilo pond-meters.

3. If you push a 10 kg weight up a vertical distance of 5 meters, the work performed would be
   a. 2 kilo pond-meters.
   b. 50 joules.
   c. 2 joules.
   d. 50 kilo pond-meters.

4. The units used for power are
   a. Newtons or kilo pond-meters per second.
   b. joules or kilo pond-meters.
   c. watts or kilo pond-meters per second.
   d. Newton-meters or joules per second.

5. How much power would it take to complete the task described in question 3 in 5 seconds?
   c. 10 joules per second
   d. 0.2 kilo pond-meters per second
   c. 10 kilo pond-meters per second
   d. 0.2 joules per second

6. The work performed by a 50 kg girl stepping up and down a 0.4 meter bench for 5 minutes at 30 steps per minute is
   a. 3000 kilo pond-meters.
   b. 3000 joules.
   c. 1.2 kilo pond-meters.
   d. 1.2 kilo joules.

7. The power output of the girl in question 6 is
   a. 600 watts.
   b. 600 kilo pond-meters per minute.
   c. 7 watts.
   d. 7 watts per minute.

8. What is the work output of 20 minutes of bicycle ergometry at 60 rpm, with a resistance of 2 Kg and the distance traveled per revolution being 6 meters?
   a. 7200 kilo pond-meters.
   b. 7200 joules.
   c. 14400 kilo pond-meters.
   d. none of the above.

9. The power output of the previous problem is
   a. 1440 kilo pond-meters per minute.
   b. 720 kilo pond-meters per minute.
   c. 1440 watts.
   d. 720 watts.

10. It is not possible to calculate the work performed on a treadmill while
    a. the treadmill is on an incline.
    b. the incline is less than 10%.
    c. the treadmill is horizontal .
    d. None of the above.

11. The work performed by an 80 kg subject running for 5 minutes on a treadmill that is traveling at 300 meters per minute at an incline of 7.5% is
    a. 112.5 kilo joules.
    b. 112.5 joules.
    c. 112.5 kilo pond-meters.
    d. 9000 kilo pond-meters.

12. The power output of the previous problem is
    a. 1800 kilo pond-meters per minute.
    b. 1800 kilojoules per minute.
    c. 22.5 watts.
    d. 22.5 kilo pond-meters per minute.

13. Direct calorimetry measures
    a. metabolic rate through oxygen consumption.
    b. metabolic rate through heat production.
    c. oxygen consumption with open circuit spirometry.
    d. oxygen consumption with closed circuit spirometry.

14. The energy liberated when fat is metabolized is
    a. 5.05 kcal.
    b. 19.7 kcal.
    c. 4.7 kcal.
    d. 21.13 kcal.

15. The energy liberated when carbohydrate is metabolized is
    a. 5.05 kcal.
    b. 19.7 kcal.
    c. 4.7 kcal.
    d. 21.13 kcal.

16. The caloric expenditure as a result of the metabolism of 1 Liter of O_2 is approximately
    a. 5 kcal.
    b. 21 Kj.
    c. 21 kcal.
    d. Both a and b are correct.

17. A person exercising at an oxygen consumption of 5.0 liters/min. would expend around
    a. 10 kcal/min.
    b. 1 kcal/min.
    c. 17.5 kcal/min.
    d. 25 kcal/min.

18. The most common technique used to measure energy expenditure uses
    a. a calorimeter.
    b. the energy of the foods eaten.
    c. closed circuit spirometry.
    d. open circuit spirometry.

19. The resting VO_2 of an individual is approximately
    a. 35 ml/kg/min.
    b. 3.5 ml/kg/min.
    c. 10 Mets.
    d. 3.5 Mets.

20. The VO_2 requirement for a 40 kg girl performing a 5 MET activity would be
    a. 0.7 liters/min.
    b. 1.4 liters/min.
    c. 0.5 liters/min.
    d. None of the above.

21. Net efficiency is defined as the ratio of
    a. work output to resting energy expenditure.
    b. work output to energy expenditure above rest.
    c. resting energy expenditure to work output.
    d. energy expenditure above rest to work output.

22. The efficiency of exercise is influenced by
    a. exercise work rate.
    b. speed of movement.
    c. fiber composition of muscles performing the exercise.
    d. All of the above.

23. Net efficiency is defined as the ratio of
    a. work output to resting energy expenditure.
    b. work output to energy expenditure above rest.
    c. resting energy expenditure to work output.
    d. energy expenditure above rest to work output.

24. A difference in efficiency between muscle fibers is due to
    a. different size of the fibers.
    b. different requirements in ATP per unit of work.
    c. different requirements in substrate per unit of work.
    d. All of the above.

25. The relationship between work rate and energy expenditure is
    a. exponential.
    b. linear.
    c. curvilinear.
    d. inverse.

True and False

Instructions: Read each question carefully and determine if the statement is true or false. The correct answers to this exam are provided at the end of the chapter.

1. The SI unit for Energy is the joule.

2. The term ergometry is associated with the measurement of work output.

3. The concept of power is important since it describes the rate at which work is being performed .

4. Quantifiable work is performed when a subject is walking or running horizontally.

5. A 10% grade indicates that for every 1 meter a subject travels horizontally he or she travels 10 meters vertically.

6. The vertical displacement of a subject traveling on a treadmill is calculated by multiplying the horizontal distance by the sine of the percent grade.

7. When the body uses energy to do work heat is released.

8. The rate of body heat production is inversely proportional to the metabolic rate.

9. In order to convert the amount of O_2 consumed into heat equivalents it is necessary to know the type of nutrient that was metabolized.

10. Open circuit spirometry measures the volume of oxygen inspired and expired.

11. It is possible to estimate energy expenditure during walking or running with reasonable precision.

12. The relationship between the oxygen cost of walking is linear, however, running is alinear.

13. Net efficiency for humans exercising on a cycle ergometer ranges from 50-60%.

14. To calculate net efficiency both the work output and power output are required.

15. VO_2 measurements to calculate efficiency must be made during steady state.

16. To calculate the net efficiency both the numerator and denominator need to be in similar terms.

17. Resting energy expenditure accounts for only a small portion of energy expenditure at low work rates.

18. There is an optimum speed of movement for any given work rate.

19. A runner who exhibits poor running economy would require a higher VO_2 at a given running speed.

20. Running economy at slow speeds is comparable between highly trained men and women.

21. Optimum speed of movement increases as the power output increases.

22. One Met is equal to resting oxygen consumption.

23. Exercise efficiency is greater in people with more slow fibers.

24. Fast fibers are more efficient than slow fibers.

25. It is possible to compute efficiency during horizontal treadmill running.

Matching Terms and Definitions

Instructions: Consider each term carefully and select the correct definition below. The correct answers are provided at the end of the chapter.

Terms
1. absolute oxygen
2. cycle ergometer
3. direct calorimetry
4. ergometer
5. ergometry
6. indirect calorimetry
7. kilo calorie (kcal)
8. MET
9. net efficiency
10. open-circuit spirometry
11. percent grade
12. power
13. relative VO_2
14. SI units
15. work

Definitions
a. Estimation of heat or energy production on the basis of oxygen consumption, carbon dioxide production and nitrogen excretion.
b. Measurement of work output.
c. Indirect calorimetry procedure in which either inspired or expired ventilation is measured and oxygen consumption and carbon dioxide production is calculated.
d. A rate of work.
e. Oxygen consumption expressed per unit body weight.
f. The amount of oxygen consumed over a given time period; expressed as L/min.

g. The product of a force and the distance through which that force moves.
h. An expression of the rate of energy expenditure at rest.
i. A stationary exercise cycle that allows accurate measurement of work output.
j. A measure of the elevation of the treadmill.
k. Instrument for measuring work.
l. A measurement of energy expenditure.
m. System used to provide international standardization of units of measure in science.
n. A simple measure of exercise efficiency defined as the ratio of work performed to energy expended above rest.
o. Assessment of the body's metabolic rate by direct measurement of the amount of heat produced.

Answers

Multiple choice		True and False		Terms and Definitions	
1.	d	1.	True	1.	f
2.	b	2.	True	2.	i
3.	c	3.	True	3.	o
4.	b	4.	False	4.	k
5.	c	5.	False	5.	b
6.	a	6.	False	6.	a
7.	b	7.	True	7.	l
8.	c	8.	False	8.	h
9.	b	9.	True	9.	n
10.	c	10.	True	10.	c
11.	d	11.	True	11.	j
12.	a	12.	False	12.	d
13.	b	13.	False	13.	e
14.	c	14.	False	14.	m
15.	a	15.	True	15.	g
16.	a	16.	True		
17.	d	17.	False		
18.	d	18.	True		
19.	b	19.	True		
20.	a	20.	True		
21.	b	21.	True		
22.	d	22.	True		
23.	b	23.	True		
24.	b	24.	False		
25.	c	25.	False		

Chapter 7: The Nervous System : Structure and Control of Movement

Chapter Learning Objectives

After studying this chapter you should be able to do the following:

1. Discuss the general organization of the nervous system.
2. Describe the structure and function of a nerve.
3. Draw and label the pathways involved in a withdrawal reflex.
4. Define depolarization, action potential, and repolarization.
5. Discuss the role of position receptors in the control of movement.
6. Describe the role of the vestibular apparatus in maintaining equilibrium.
7. Discuss the brain centers involved in voluntary control of movement.
8. Describe the structure and function of the autonomic nervous system.

Multiple Choice

Instructions: After reading the question, and all possible answers, select the letter of choice that *BEST* answers the question. *Read all possible answers because some questions may have more than one correct answer.* The correct answers are provided at the end of this chapter.

1. The nervous system is divided into two major divisions
   a. central and parasympathetic.
   b. autonomic and peripheral.
   c. central and autonomic.
   d. central and peripheral.

2. The following is true of a sensory fiber
   a. conduct information towards the CNS.
   b. are known as efferent fibers.
   c. innervate involuntary effector organs only.
   d. Both a and b are correct.

3. The axon carries the electrical message
   a. towards the nerve cell.
   b. away from the nerve cell.
   c. to the CNS.
   d. none of the above.

4. The discontinuous sheath that covers the outside of axons are
   a. Schwann cells.
   b. nodes of Ranvier.
   c. dendrites.
   d. neurofibrils.

5. The resting membrane potential of a neuron is generally
   a. -40 to -75 mv.
   b. 40 to 70 mv.
   c. approximately 100 mv.
   d. approximately -200 mv.

6. What mechanism ensures that there is little change in resting membrane potential?
   a. the diffusion of sodium into the cell.
   b. the diffusion of potassium out of the cell.
   c. sodium/potassium pump.
   d. All of the above.

7. The first stage of the generation of a neural message is
   a. the formation of an action potential.
   b. the change in polarity to become more negative.
   c. the entry of potassium into the cell.
   d. the entry of sodium into the cell.

8. Neurotransmitters that cause depolarization of membranes are called
   a. inhibitory transmitters.
   b. receptors.
   c. excitatory transmittors.
   d. none of the above.

9. The summing of several EPSP's from a single pre synaptic neuron over a short time period is called
   a. spatial summation.
   b. temporal summation.
   c. IPSP.
   d. hyper polarization.

10. An example of proprioreceptors that provide the CNS with information are
    a. muscle spindles.
    b. golgi tendon organs.
    c. joint receptors.
    d. all of the above.

11. The withdrawal reflex results in
    a. contraction of extensor muscles on the side stimulated.
    b. contraction of flexor muscles on the side stimulated.
    c. inhibition of extensor muscles on the side not stimulated.
    d. None of the above.

12. The storage of learned motor experiences is performed by the
    a. cerebellum.
    b. cerebrum.
    c. pons.
    d. medulla.

13. Evidence exists to suggest that the control of movement in response to feedback from proprioceptors is carried out by the
    a. cerebellum.
    b. cerebrum.
    c. pons.
    d. medulla.

14. The first step in performing a voluntary movement is thought to occur in the
    a. cerebellum.
    b. brain stem.
    c. sub cortical and cortical areas.
    d. basal ganglia.

15. The sympathetic division of the autonomic nervous system has it's preganglionic cell bodies in
    a. brain stem and sacral spinal cord.
    b. brain stem and thoracic spinal cord.
    c. thoracic spinal cord and lumbar spinal cord.
    d. lumbar spinal cord and sacral spinal cord.

16. The neurotransmitter released at the effector organ by the sympathetic nervous system
    is primarily
    a. acetylcholine.
    b. epinephrine.
    c. insulin.
    d. norepinephrine.

17. Repolarization occurs due to
    a. increased permeability to potassium.
    b. decreased permeability to sodium.
    c. decreased permeability to potassium.
    d. Both a and b are correct.

18. Synaptic transmission occurs when
    a. decreased neuronal permeability to sodium.
    b. increased neuronal permeability to potassium.
    c. sufficient amounts of neurotransmittors are released.
    d. All of the above.

19. The maintenance of the body's internal environment is carried out by the
    a. parasympathetic nervous system.
    b. sympathetic nervous system.
    c. autonomic nervous system.
    d. All of the above.

20. The motor cortex controls motor activity with the aid of input from the
    a. subcortical areas.
    b. cerebral cortex.
    c. cerebrum.
    d. motor units.

True and False

Instructions: Read each question carefully and determine if the statement is true or false. The correct answers to this exam are provided at the end of the chapter.

1. The somatic motor portion of the peripheral nervous system innervates skeletal muscle.

2. The axon of a neuron contains dendrites.

3. The net charge on the outside of a membrane is negative.

4. At rest, sodium concentration is much greater outside the cell than inside.

5. At rest, the sodium gates are open much wider than the potassium gates.

6. Repolarization occurs due to potassium entering the cell.

7. If a nerve impulse is initiated, the impulse will travel the entire length of the axon.
   without a decrease in voltage

8. A common neurotransmitter at the nerve/muscle junction is acetylcholine.

9. The end result of an IPSP is hypo polarization.

10. Reflex contraction of skeletal muscles is not dependent on the activation of higher brain centers.

11. The maintenance of balance is due to feedback concerning the position of the eyes.

12. The portion of the brain most concerned with voluntary movement is the motor cortex.

13. Feedback to the CNS from muscle and joint receptors allow for adjustment to improve the movement pattern.

14. The autonomic nervous system involves somatic motor nerves.

15. Most organs receive innervation from only one division of the autonomic nervous system.

16. At rest neurons are negatively charged outside the cell with respect to the inside.

17. The gaps between Schwann cells are called dendrites.

18. Pacinian corpuscles are position receptors.

19. The somatic neuron that innervates skeletal muscle is called a motor neuron.

20. Control of voluntary movement is complex and requires the co-operation of many areas of the brain.

Matching Terms and Definitions

Instructions: Consider each term carefully and select the correct definition below. The correct answers are provided at the end of the chapter.

Terms and Definitions (Group 1)

Terms (Group 1)
1. action potential
2. afferent fibers
3. autonomic nervous system
4. axon
5. brain stem
6. cell body
7. central nervous system
8. cerebellum
9. cerebrum
10. conductivity
11. dendrites
12. efferent fibers
13. EPSP
14. IPSP
15. irritability

Definitions (Group 1)
a. Capacity for conduction.
b. Portion of the brain that includes mid brain, pons and medulla.
c. A graded depolarization of a post-synaptic membrane by a neurotransmitter.
d. The all or none electrical event in the neuron or muscle cell in which the polarity of the cell membrane is rapidly reversed and re-established.
e. A trait of certain tissues that enables them to respond to stimuli.
f. Superior aspect of the brain that occupies the upper cranial cavity.
g. Portion of the brain that is concerned with fine co-ordination of skeletal muscles during movement.
h. Moves the post synaptic membrane further from threshold.
i. Portion of the nerve fiber that transmits action potentials toward a nerve cell body.
j. Portion of the nervous system that functions to control the actions of visceral organs.

k. Nerve fibers that carry neural information from the central nervous system to the periphery.
l. The major portion of the body of a nerve cell.
m. Portion of the nervous system that consists of the brain and spinal cord.
n. A nerve fiber that conducts a nerve impulse away from the neuron cell body.
o. Nerve fibers that carry neural information back to the central nervous system.

Terms and Definitions (Group 2)

Terms (Group 2)

1. kinesthesia
2. motor cortex
3. neuron
4. parasympathetic nervous system
5. peripheral nervous system
6. proprioceptors
7. reciprocal inhibition
8. resting membrane potential
9. Schwann cells
10. spatial summation
11. sympathetic nervous system
12. synapses
13. temporal summation
14. vestibular apparatus

Definitions (Group 2)

a. Composed of a cell body with dendrites that bring information to the cell body and axons that take information away from the cell body.
b. Portion of the nervous system located outside the spinal cord and brain.
c. A change in the membrane potential produced by the addition of two or more inputs occurring at different times.
d. Sensory organ that provides needed information about body position to maintain balance.
e. A perception of movement obtained from information about the position and rate of movement of a joint.
f. Portion of the autonomic nervous system that primarily releases acetylcholine from it's post-ganglionic nerve endings.
g. The additive effect of numerous simultaneous inputs to different sites on a neuron to produce a change in the membrane potential.
h. The cell that surrounds peripheral nerve fibers forming the myelin sheath.
i. Portion of the autonomic nervous system that releases norepinephrine.
j. Portion of the cerebral cortex containing large motor units whose axons descend to lower brain centers and spinal cord; associated with voluntary movement.
k. The voltage difference measured across a membrane that is related to the concentration of ions on each side of the membrane and the permeability of the membrane to those ions.
l. When extensor muscles are contracted there is a reflex inhibition of the motor neurons to the flexor muscles and vice-versa.
m. Receptors that provide information about the position and movement of the body.
n. Junctions between nerve cells where the electrical activity of one neuron influences another neuron.

Answers

Multiple Choice

1. d
2. a
3. b
4. a
5. a
6. c
7. d
8. c
9. b
10. d
11. b
12. b
13. a
14. c
15. c
16. d
17. d
18. c
19. c
20. a

True and False

1. True
2. False
3. False
4. True
5. False
6. False
7. True
8. True
9. False
10. True
11. False
12. True
13. True
14. False
15. False
16. False
17. False
18. True
19. True
20. True

Terms and Definitions (Group 1)

1. d
2. o
3. j
4. n
5. b
6. l
7. m
8. g
9. f
10. a
11. i
12. k
13. c
14. h
15. e

Terms and Definitions (Group 2)

1. e
2. j
3. a
4. f
5. b
6. m
7. l
8. k
9. h
10. g
11. i
12. n
13. c
14. d

Chapter 8: Skeletal Muscle

Chapter Learning Objectives

After studying this chapter you should be able to do the following:

1. Draw and label the micro structure of skeletal muscle.
2. Outline the steps leading to muscle contraction.
3. Define the terms *isotonic* and *isometric*.
4. Discuss the following terms: 1) *simple twitch*, 2) *summation*, and 3) *tetanus*.
5. Discuss the major biochemical and mechanical properties of the three human skeletal fiber types.
6. Discuss the relationship between skeletal muscle fiber types and performance.
7. List and discuss those factors that regulate the amount of force exerted during muscular contraction.
8. Graph the relationship between movement velocity and the amount of force exerted during muscular contraction.
9. Discuss the structure and function of a muscle spindle.
10. Describe the function of a Golgi tendon organ.

Multiple Choice

Instructions: After reading the question, and all possible answers, select the letter of choice that *BEST* answers the question. *Read all possible answers because some questions may have more than one correct answer.* The correct answers are provided at the end of this chapter.

1. The striated appearance of skeletal muscle is due to
   a. being multinucleated.
   b. arrangement of actin and myosin.
   c. overlap of the I band and the H zone.
   d. the Z lines.

2. Sarcomeres are divided from each other by
   a. Z lines.
   b. A bands.
   c. I bands.
   d. H zones.

3. Muscle fibers contract by shortening of their
   a. myofibrils.
   b. Z line to Z line distance.
   c. A bands.
   d. Both a and b are correct.

4. The energy for muscular contraction comes from
   a. the release of acetylcholine.
   b. the pulling of actin over the myosin molecule.
   c. the breakdown of ATP by myosin ATPase.
   d. None of the above.

5. Muscle fibers with a relatively small number of mitochondria are
   a. Fast-twitch fibers
   b. Slow-twitch fibers
   c. Intermediate fibers
   d. Type I fibers

6. The red pigment of type I fibers is due to
   a. hemoglobin.
   b. myoglobin.
   c. mitochondria.
   d. All of the above.

7. The predominant muscle fiber of non-athletes is
   a. type I.
   b. type IIa.
   c. type II.
   d. None of the above.

8. Endurance training results in conversion of muscle fibers from
   a. type I to type IIa.
   b. type IIa to type II.
   c. type I to type II.
   d. type II to type I.

9. A contraction where a muscle exerts tension but does not shorten in length is an
   a. isometric contraction.
   b. isotonic contraction.
   c. isokinetic contraction.
   d. eccentric contraction.

10. The amount of force generated by a muscle fiber depends primarily on
    a. the stimulation.
    b. number of actin/myosin cross bridges in contact.
    c. a decreased latent period.
    d. Both a and b are correct.

11. The amount of force generated by a group of muscles depends on
    a. type and number of motor units recruited.
    b. initial length of the muscle.
    c. nature of the neural stimulation.
    d. All of the above.

12. Muscular contractions are stimulated by
    a. single twitches.
    b. alternate twitches.
    c. addition of successive twitches.
    d. None of the above.

13. The loss of muscle mass in aging humans is often due to
    a. increased activity levels.
    b. hypertrophy due to hormonal changes.
    c. atrophy due to disuse.
    d. a shift in fiber type.

14. From age 25 to 50 years the muscle mass lost is around
    a. 5%.
    b. 10%.
    c. 20%.
    d. 50%.

15. The muscle spindle acts directly on the
    a. tendon.
    b. joint.
    c. central nervous system.
    d. muscle.

16. When comparing contractile properties of muscle fibers which characteristic(s) is/are important
    a. maximal force production.
    b. speed of contraction.
    c. muscle fiber efficiency.
    d. All of the above.

17. Type IIb fibers have
    a. a large number of mitochondria.
    b. limited capacity for aerobic metabolism.
    c. limited glycolytic capacity.
    d. None of the above.

18. In the resting state the myosin cross-bridges
    a. remain connected to actin in a weak binding state.
    b. remain connected to actin in a strong binding state.
    c. are not connected to actin.
    d. are bound to troponin.

19. The contraction cycle can continue as long as there is
    a. calcium present.
    b. ATP present.
    c. ADP present.
    d. Both a and b are correct.

20. During excitation contraction-coupling calcium binds to
    a. actin.
    b. tropomyosin.
    c. troponin.
    d. myosin.

True and False

Instructions: Read each question carefully and determine if the statement is true or false. The correct answers to this exam are provided at the end of the chapter.

1. Muscle cells have the same organelles as found in other cells.

2. The transverse tubules are the storage site for Ca^{++}.

3. The binding of acetylcholine on the motor end plate causes a decrease in the permeability of the sarcolemma to sodium.

4. Calcium is released from the sarcoplasmic reticulum and binds with tropomyosin.

5. Thyroxine is a powerful regulator of muscle fiber type.

6. The rate at which action potentials are conducted along the motor neurons that innervate slow twitch fibers is slower than that of fast twitch fibers.

7. It is the motor neuron that determines the characteristic of the muscle fiber at the other end.

8. Inactivity of muscles causes a type II muscle fiber to become slower.

9. Skeletal muscle is capable of changing it's biochemical makeup.

10. Slow twitch fibers exert more force than fast twitch fibers.

11. There is an ideal length of a muscle fiber for optimum force generation.

12. Increasing the stimulus to activate more motor units does not result in an increased force generation.

13. The power produced by a muscle group decreases as the velocity of movement increases.

14. Golgi tendon organs provide feedback about the length of the muscle.

15. Muscle spindles are innervated by gamma motor neurons which detect tension development.

16. Type I fibers possess a faster shortening velocity than type IIb fibers.

17. Fast fibers have a higher maximal force production than slow fibers.

18. Muscular contraction occurs by multiple cycles of cross-bridge activity.

19. Troponin covers the active sites on actin.

20. Biochemical and contractile properties of the different muscle fibers represent a continuum.

Matching Terms and Definitions

Instructions: Consider each term carefully and select the correct definition below. The correct answers are provided at the end of the chapter.

Terms and Definitions (Group 1)

Terms (Group 1)
1. actin
2. concentric contraction
3. dynamic
4. eccentric contraction
5. endomycium
6. end-plate potential (EPP)
7. epimycium
8. extensors
9. fasciculi
10. fast twitch fibers
11. flexors
12. golgi tendon organs
13. intermediate fibers
14. isometric
15. isotonic
16. lateral sac
17. motor neurons
18. motor unit
19. muscle spindle

Definitions (Group 1)

a. A contraction in which the muscle develops tension but does not shorten.
b. Muscle fiber type that generates high force at a moderately fast speed of contraction but has a relatively large number of mitochondria.
c. A small bundle of muscle fibers.
d. A structural protein of muscle that works with myosin permitting muscular contraction.
e. Depolarization of a membrane region by a sodium influx.
f. Refers to an isotonic muscle contraction.
g. Muscles that function to extend the limb.
h. A muscle stretch receptor.
i. One of several types of muscle fibers found in skeletal muscle also called type II fibers.
j. A tension receptor located in series with skeletal muscle.
k. A motor neuron and all the muscle fibers innervated by that single motor neuron.
l. Efferent neurons that conduct action potentials from the CNS to the muscles.
m. When a muscle is activated and shortens.
n. Contraction in which a muscle shortens against a constant load or tension resulting in movement.
o. The outer layer of connective tissue surrounding muscle.
p. Muscle groups that cause flexion of limbs.
q. The inner layer of connective tissue surrounding a muscle fiber.
r. When a muscle is activated and lengthens.
s. Where stored calcium is released from.

Terms and Definitions (Group 2)

Terms (Group 2)

1. myofibrils
2. myosin
3. neuromuscular junction
4. perimycium
5. sarcolemma
6. sarcomeres
7. sarcoplasmic reticulum
8. sliding filament model
9. slow twitch fibers
10. static
11. summation
12. terminal cisternae
13. tetanus
14. transverse tubules
15. tropomyosin
16. troponin
17. type I fibers
18. type IIa fibers
19. type IIb fibers
20. twitch

Definitions (Group 2)

a. Muscle fiber type that contracts slowly.
b. Describes a muscle contraction in which tension is developed, but the muscle does not shorten.
c. Portion of a muscle containing thick and thin contractile filaments.
d. Protein associated with actin and tropomyosin that binds calcium and initiates the movement of tropomyosin on actin.
e. The cell membrane surrounding a muscle fiber.
f. Slow twitch fibers that contain large numbers of oxidative enzymes.
g. An extension of the muscle membrane that conducts the action potential into the muscle to depolarize the terminal cisternae.
h. Highest tension developed by a muscle in response to a high frequency of stimulation.
i. Portion of the sarcoplasmic reticulum near the transverse tubule containing the Ca^{++} that is released upon depolarization of the muscle.
j. Contractile protein in the thick filament of a myofibril that contains the cross bridge that can bind actin and split ATP to cause tension development.

k. Synapse between axon terminal of a motor neuron and the motor end plate of a muscles plasma membrane.
l. Repeated stimulation of a muscle that leads to an increase in tension compared to a single twitch.
m. Protein covering the actin binding sites that prevents the myosin cross bridge from touching actin.
n. The repeated contractile unit in a myofibril, bounded by Z lines.
o. A membrane structure that surrounds the myofibrils of muscle cells, location of the terminal cisternae.
p. The tension generated response following the application of a single stimulus to muscle.
q. A model of muscle contraction.
r. Connective tissue surrounding the fasiculus.
s. Fast twitch fibers that have a relatively small number of mitochondria.
t. Intermediate fibers also known as fast-oxidative glycolytic fibers.

Answers

Multiple Choice
1. b
2. a
3. d
4. c
5. a
6. b
7. d
8. d
9. a
10. b
11. d
12. c
13. c
14. b
15. c
16. d
17. b
18. a
19. d
20. c

True and False
1. True
2. False
3. False
4. False
5. True
6. True
7. True
8. False
9. True
10. False
11. True
12. False
13. False
14. False
15. False
16. False
17. True
18. True
19. False
20. True

Terms and Definitions (Group 1)
1. d
2. m
3. f
4. r
5. q
6. e
7. o
8. g
9. c
10. i
11. p
12. j
13. b
14. a
15. n
16. s
17. l
18. k
19. h

Terms and Definitions (Group 2)

1.	c		11.	l
2.	j		12.	i
3.	k		13.	h
4.	r		14.	g
5.	e		15.	m
6.	n		16.	d
7.	o		17.	f
8.	q		18.	s
9.	a		19.	t
10.	b		20.	p

Chapter 9: Circulatory Adaptations to Exercise

Chapter Learning Objectives

After studying this chapter you should be able to do the following:

1. Give an overview of the design and function of the circulatory system.
2. Describe the cardiac cycle and the associated electrical activity recorded via the electrocardiogram.
3. Discuss the pattern of redistribution of blood flow during exercise.
4. Outline the circulatory responses to various types of exercise.
5. Identify the factors that regulate local blood flow during exercise.
6. List and discuss those factors responsible for regulation of stroke volume during exercise.
7. Discuss the regulation of cardiac output during exercise.

Multiple Choice

Instructions: After reading the question, and all possible answers, select the letter of choice that *BEST* answers the question. *Read all possible answers because some questions may have more than one correct answer.* The correct answers are provided at the end of this chapter.

1. Back flow from the arteries into the ventricles is prevented by the
   a. atrioventricular valves.
   b. tricuspid valves.
   c. semilunar valves.
   d. bicuspid valves.

2. Oxygenated blood returns to the heart via the
   a. pulmonary artery.
   b. pulmonary vein.
   c. superior vena cava.
   d. aorta.

3. At rest, contraction of the ventricles ejects about
   a. one third of the blood.
   b. two thirds of the blood.
   c. half of the blood.
   d. None of the above.

4. Increases in heart rate during exercise are achieved primarily through
   a. an increase in the time spent in diastole.
   b. an increase in the time spent in systole.
   c. an decrease in the time spent in systole.
   d. an decrease in the time spent in diastole.

5. The P wave of an ECG results from
   a. atrial depolarization.
   b. atrial repolarization.
   c. ventricular repolarization.
   d. ventricular depolarization.

6. Cardiac output can be increased with a rise in
   a. heart rate.
   b. stroke volume.
   c. ST segment of the ECG.
   d. Both a and b are correct.

7. The major influence on end diastolic volume is
   a. strength of ventricular contraction.
   b. lengthening of cardiac fibers.
   c. venous return.
   d. afterload.

8. The determinant/s of heart rate are
   a. parasympathetic nervous system.
   b. sympathetic nervous system.
   c. cardiac output.
   d. Both a and b are correct.

9. The average hematocrit of a normal male is approximately
   a. 42%.
   b. 97%.
   c. 49%.
   d. 21%.

10. Stroke volume does not increase beyond a workload of approximately _____ VO_2 max.
    a. 60%
    b. 40%
    c. 20%
    d. 80%

11. The a-v O_2 difference represents
    a. cardiac output.
    b. stroke volume.
    c. O_2 uptake by the tissues.
    d. Both a and b are correct.

12. During maximal exercise _____ of total cardiac output is directed to contracting skeletal muscle.
    a. 15%-20%
    b. 100%
    c. 60%-65%
    d. 80%-85%

13. During exercise, vascular resistance to visceral organs increases due to
    a. increased adrenergic sympathetic output.
    b. decreased adrenergic sympathetic output.
    c. increased parasympathetic activity.
    d. None of the above.

14. Cardiovascular drift is due to
    a. decrease in heart rate.
    b. increase in stroke volume.
    c. cutaneous vasoconstriction.
    d. None of the above.

50

15. The initial signal to the cardiovascular system at the onset of exercise comes from
    a. baroreceptors.
    b. chemoreceptors.
    c. higher brain centers.
    d. All of the above.

16. Baroreceptors are sensitive to changes in
    a. muscle metabolites.
    b. muscle pressure.
    c. arterial pressure.
    d. None of the above.

17. The increased metabolic demand placed on the heart during exercise can be best estimated by examining the
    a. double product.
    b. systolic blood pressure.
    c. diastolic blood pressure.
    d. heart rate.

18. Oxygen delivery to exercising skeletal muscle increases due to
    a. decreased cardiac output.
    b. redistribution of blood flow to inactive organs.
    c. decrease in arterial blood pressure.
    d. none of the above.

19. The release of nitric oxide promotes
    a. smooth muscle relaxation.
    b. vasodilation.
    c. increased blood flow.
    d. All of the above.

20. Endurance athletes have improved ventricular filling due to
    a. decreased heart rate.
    b. increased venous return.
    c. decreased venous return.
    d. decreased stroke volume.

True and False

Instructions: Read each question carefully and determine if the statement is true or false. The correct answers to this exam are provided at the end of the chapter.

1. Mixed venous blood is returned to the left side of the heart.

2. The myocardium receives its blood supply via the left and right coronary arteries.

3. Heart muscle contains actin and myosin myofilaments.

4. Systolic blood pressure is produced as blood is ejected from the heart during ventricular relaxation.

5. Myocardial cells have the unique potential for spontaneous electrical activity.

6. A release in acetylcholine causes a decrease in the activity of the SA and AV nodes.

7. Stimulation of the SA and AV nodes by the parasympathetic nervous system is responsible for increases in heart rate.

8. The flow of blood is proportional to the resistance.

9. The greatest vascular resistance occurs in the arterioles.

10. Cardiac output increases during exercise in direct proportion to the required metabolic rate.

11. As exercise progresses vasodilation can be maintained by intrinsic regulation.

12. Changes in heart rate and blood pressure during exercise do not depend on the intensity of the exercise.

13. The increase in cardiac output during incremental exercise is achieved by a decrease in arterial blood pressure.

14. Heart rate is higher during leg exercise compared to arm exercise.

15. With prolonged exercise heart rate declines while stroke volume increases.

16. Fine-tuning of the cardiovascular responses are carried out by baroreceptors.

17. The greatest vascular resistance to blood flow is offered in the capillaries

18. The most important factor determining resistance to blood flow is the radius of the blood vessel.

19. Stroke volume does not plateau in endurance athletes.

20. Cardiovascular adjustments at the beginning of exercise are slow.

Matching Terms and Definitions

Instructions: Consider each term carefully and select the correct definition below. The correct answers are provided at the end of the chapter.

Terms
1. arteries
2. arterioles
3. atrioventricular node (AV node)
4. autoregulation
5. capillaries
6. cardiac accelerator nerves
7. cardiac output
8. cardiovascular control center
9. central command
10. diastole
11. diastolic blood pressure
12. double product
13. electrocardiogram
14. intercalated discs
15. mixed venous blood
16. myocardium
17. pulmonary circuit
18. sinoatrial node
19. stroke volume
20. systole
21. systolic blood pressure
22. vagus nerve
23. veins
24. venules

Definitions

a. Arterial blood pressure during diastole.
b. The amount of blood pumped by the heart per unit of time.
c. Portion of the cardiovascular system involved in the circulation of blood from the heart to the lungs and back to the heart.
d. Amount of blood pumped by the ventricles in a single beat.
e. Part of the sympathetic nervous system that stimulates the SA node to increase heart rate.
f. Blood vessels that accepts blood from the venules and brings it back to the heart.
g. Mechanism by which an organ regulates blood flow to match the metabolic rate.
h. Large vessels that carry arterialized blood away from the heart.
i. Cardiac muscle.
j. A mixture of venous blood from both the upper and lower extremities.
k. Period of filling of the heart between contractions.
l. A small branch of an artery that communicates with a capillary network.
m. Small blood vessels carrying capillary blood to veins.
n. Functions in the transmission of cardiac impulses from the atria to the ventricles.
o. Portion of the cardiac cycle in which the ventricles are contracting.
p. Control of the cardiovascular or pulmonary system by cortical impulses.
q. Portion of cardiac muscle cell where one cell connects to the next.
r. Major parasympathetic nerve.
s. Microscopic blood vessels that connect arterioles and venules.
t. Generates the electrical impulse to initiate the heart beat.
u. Highest arterial pressure measured during the cardiac cycle.
v. Recording of electrical changes that occur in the myocardium.
w. The area of the medulla that regulates the cardiovascular system.
x. The product of the heart rate and the systolic pressure.

Answers

Multiple choice		True and False		Terms and Definitions	
1.	c	1.	False	1.	h
2.	b	2.	True	2.	l
3.	b	3.	True	3.	n
4.	d	4.	False	4.	g
5.	a	5.	True	5.	s
6.	d	6.	True	6.	e
7.	c	7.	False	7.	b
8.	d	8.	False	8.	w
9.	a	9.	True	9.	p
10.	b	10.	True	10.	k
11.	c	11.	True	11.	a
12.	d	12.	False	12.	x
13.	a	13.	False	13.	v
14.	d	14.	False	14.	q
15.	c	15.	False	15.	j
16.	c	16.	False	16.	i
17.	a	17.	False	17.	c
18.	d	18.	True	18.	t
19.	d	19.	True	19.	d
20.	b	20.	False	20.	o
				21.	u
				22.	r
				23.	f
				24.	m

Chapter 10: Respiration During Exercise

Chapter learning objectives

After studying this chapter you should be able to do the following:

1. Explain the principal physiological function of the pulmonary system.
2. Outline the major anatomical components of the respiratory system.
3. List the major muscles involved in inspiration and expiration at rest and during exercise.
4. Discuss the importance of matching blood flow to alveolar ventilation in the lung.
5. Explain how gases are transported across the blood-gas interface in the lung.
6. Discuss the major transportation modes of O_2 and CO_2 in the blood.
7. Discuss the effects of increasing temperature, decreasing pH, and increasing levels of 2-3 DPG on the oxygen-hemoglobin dissociation curve.
8. Describe the ventilatory response to constant load steady state exercise. What happens to ventilation if exercise is prolonged and performed in a high-temperature/humid environment?
9. Describe the ventilatory response to incremental exercise. What factors are thought to contribute to the alinear rise in ventilation at work rates above 50%-70% of O_2 max?
10. Identify the location and function of chemoreceptors and mechanoreceptors that are thought to play a role in the regulation of breathing.
11. Discuss the neural-humoral theory of respiratory control during exercise.

Multiple Choice

Instructions: After reading the question, and all possible answers, select the letter of choice that *BEST* answers the question. *Read all possible answers because some questions may have more than one correct answer.* The correct answers are provided at the end of this chapter.

1. Cellular respiration refers to
   a. the exchange of gases at the lungs.
   b. oxygen utilization and carbon dioxide production at the tissues.
   c. pulmonary respiration.
   d. the ability of the alveolar to exchange gases at the lungs.

2. During exercise the respiratory system plays a role in acid-base balance by
   a. removing H+ from the blood by the HCO_3^- reaction.
   b. aiding the kidney in the removal of lactic acid.
   c. lowering the pH of the blood by hyperventilating.
   d. increasing the pH of the blood by hypoventilating.

3. The conducting zone of the respiratory system
   a. serves as a passageway for air.
   b. has alveoli which allows for gas exchange to occur.
   c. functions to humidify and filter the air.
   d. Both a and c are correct.

4. Expiration occurs when the pressure within the lungs exceeds atmospheric pressure and
   a. involves the contraction of the diaphragm
   b. is passive during normal quiet breathing
   c. requires contraction of the diaphragm only during exercise or voluntary hyperventilation
   d. Both b and c are correct

5. During exercise pulmonary ventilation increases due to
   a. an increase in both alveolar and dead space ventilation.
   b. an increase in alveolar ventilation and a decrease in dead space ventilation.
   c. an increase in the vital capacity.
   d. None of the above.

6. During exercise, the region of the lung that receives an increased percentage of the total ventilation is the
   a. apical regions.
   b. basal regions.
   c. alveolar regions.
   d. capillary regions.

7. Fick's law of diffusion states that the rate of gas transfer is proportional to
   a. the tissue area and the difference in the partial pressure of the gas on the two sides of the tissue.
   b. the thickness and the tissue area.
   c. the tissue area, the diffusion coefficient of the gas and the difference in the partial pressure of the gas on the two sides of the tissue.
   d. None of the above.

8. The partial pressure of oxygen is
   a. higher in the alveoli than the pulmonary artery.
   b. higher in the pulmonary artery than the systemic arteries.
   c. higher in the systemic arteries than the alveoli.
   d. higher in the systemic veins than the arteries.

9. The partial pressure of carbon dioxide is
   a. higher in the alveoli than the pulmonary artery.
   b. higher in the pulmonary artery than the systemic arteries.
   c. higher in the alveoli than the systemic arteries.
   d. higher in the systemic arteries than the veins.

10. A V/Q relationship less than 1.0 represents
    a. a greater blood flow than ventilation which is advantageous during exercise.
    b. a greater blood flow than ventilation which is disadvantageous during exercise.
    c. a greater ventilation than blood flow which is advantageous during exercise.
    d. a greater ventilation than blood flow which is disadvantageous during exercise.

11. During exercise there is a shift in the oxygen-hemoglobin dissociation curve
    a. to the right due to a decrease in pH.
    b. which allows for greater unloading of oxygen at the tissues due to an increased affinity of oxygen for hemoglobin.
    c. which allows for a increased loading of oxygen at the lungs due to a decreased affinity of oxygen for hemoglobin.
    d. All of the above.

12. Removal of CO_2 from the blood will decrease hydrogen ion concentration and thus
    a. decrease pH.
    b. increase pH.
    c. increase pH initially then decrease it.
    d. decrease pH initially then increase it.

13. Ventilation increases as a linear function of oxygen uptake up to a point known as the
    a. PCO_2 inflection point.
    b. steady state inflection point.
    c. ventilatory threshold.
    d. Both b and c are correct.

14. Input into the respiratory control center can be classified two ways
    a. pneumotaxic and apneustic.
    b. aortic and carotid.
    c. O_2 and CO_2.
    d. neural and humoral.

15. Exercise induced hypoxemia results from
    a. shift in the oxygen-hemoglobin dissociation curve.
    b. decreased VO_2 max.
    c. depressed O_2 and CO_2 receptors.
    d. pulmonary system inadequacy.

16. Central chemoreceptors are sensitive to increases in
    a. PCO_2.
    b. pH.
    c. PO_2.
    d. Both a and b are correct.

17. The likely mechanism that explains that explains the alinear rise in ventilation during an incremental exercise test is
    a. circulatory deficiency.
    b. aortic and carotid bodies are depressed.
    c. blood hydrogen ion concentration.
    d. None of the above.

18. Afferent input to the respiratory control center during exercise might come from
    a. peripheral receptors.
    b. aortic and carotid bodies.
    c. pneumotaxic area.
    d. apneustic area.

19. The depth of breathing is primarily regulated by
    a. aortic and carotid bodies.
    b. pneumotaxic and apneustic areas.
    c. O_2 and CO_2 levels.
    d. blood hydrogen ion concentration..

20. The initial drive to inspire or expire comes from neurons located in the
    a. medulla oblongata.
    b. cerebral cortex.
    c. adrenal medulla.
    d. cerebrum.

True and False

Instructions: Read each question carefully and determine if the statement is true or false. The correct answers to this exam are provided at the end of the chapter.

1. The term ventilation refers to both the mechanical process of moving air into and out of the lungs and the exchange of gases at the tissues.

2. The diaphragm is the most important muscle of inspiration and is the only skeletal muscle considered essential for life.

3. The volume of gas that reaches the respiratory zone is referred to as alveolar ventilation.

4. According to Daltons law, the total pressure of a gas mixture is equal to the sum of the barometric pressures of each gas.

5. During exercise the rate of O_2 uptake and CO_2 output may increase twenty to thirty times above resting conditions.

6. The pressures in the pulmonary circulation are relatively high when compared to those in the systemic circulation.

7. It appears that both light and heavy exercise improve the V/Q relationship.

8. An increase in temperature and pH shifts the oxygen-hemoglobin dissociation curve to the right.

9. Myoglobin has a greater affinity for oxygen than hemoglobin .

10. Carbon dioxide is transported in the blood mainly bound to hemoglobin.

11. During exercise in a hot/humid environment ventilation decreases perhaps due to an increase in body temperature affecting the respiratory control center.

12. The primary drive to increase ventilation during exercise comes from neural afferents and/or efferents.

13. The alinear rise in ventilation that occurs during a submaximal test is due to a decrease in H^+ concentration.

14. The lungs are not thought to limit performance in prolonged submaximal exercise in healthy young individuals.

15. The pulmonary system is considered to a limiting factor during prolonged submaximal exercise.

16. The peripheral chemoreceptors are the most important.

17. Exercise training does not alter the structure of the lung.

18. At the onset of constant-load submaximal exercise ventilation increases rapidly.

19. Incremental exercise results in a linear increase in ventilation up to 100% of VO_2 max.

20. Arterial PO_2 and CO_2 are maintained relatively constant during constant-load submaximal exercise.

Matching Terms and Definitions

Instructions: Consider each term carefully and select the correct definition below. The correct answers are provided at the end of the chapter.

Terms
1. alveolar ventilation
2. alveoli – o
3. anatomical dead space
4. aortic bodies
5. Bohr effect
6. bulk flow
7. carotid bodies
8. cellular respiration
9. deoxyhemoglobin – n
10. diaphragm – f
11. diffusion – Y
12. hemoglobin – M
13. myoglobin – V
14. oxyhemoglobin – J
15. partial pressure – G
16. pleura
17. pulmonary respiration
18. residual volume – R
19. respiration – Q
20. spirometry
21. tidal volume
22. total lung capacity (TLC) – X
23. ventilation – t
24. ventilatory threshold (Tvent)
25. vital capacity (VC)

Definitions
a. A thin lining of cells that is attached to the inside of the chest wall and the lung.
b. Measurement of various lung volumes.
c. The right shift of the oxyhemoglobin dissociation curve due to a decrease of blood pH.
d. Hemoglobin not in combination with oxygen.
e. The total volume of the lung (i.e., conducting airways) that does not participate in gas exchange.
f. The major respiratory muscle responsible for inspiration. Dome shaped-separates the thoracic cavity from the abdominal cavity.
g. Mass movement of molecules from an area of high pressure to an area of lower pressure.
h. Has two definitions in physiology; 1) exchange of oxygen and carbon dioxide between the lungs, 2) the use of oxygen by the cell.
i. The "breakpoint" at which pulmonary ventilation and carbon dioxide output begin to increase exponentially during an incremental exercise test.
j. Hemoglobin combined with oxygen; 1.34 ml of oxygen can combine with 1g Hb.
k. The volume of gas that reaches the alveolar region of the lung.
l. Receptors located in the arch of the aorta that are capable of detecting changes in PO_2.
m. A heme containing protein in red blood cells that is responsible for transporting oxygen to tissues. Also serves as a weak buffer within red blood cells.
n. Process of oxygen consumption and carbon dioxide production in cells (i.e., bioenergetics).
o. Microscopic air sacs located in the lung where gas exchange occurs between respiratory gases and the blood.
p. The fractional part of the barometric pressure due to the presence of a simple gas, e.g., PO_2, PCO_2 and PN_2.
q. Term that refers to ventilation (breathing) of the lung.
r. The volume of air that can be moved into and out of the lungs in one breath; equal to the sum of the inspiratory and expiratory reserve volumes and the tidal volume.
s. Chemoreceptors located in the internal carotid artery; respond to changes in PCO_2, and pH.
t. Volume of air inhaled or exhaled in a single breath.

u. The total volume of air the lung can contain; equal to the sum of the vital capacity and the residual volume.

v. Protein in muscle that can bind oxygen and release it at low PO_2 values; aids in the diffusion of oxygen from capillary to mitochondria.

w. The movement of air into and out of the lungs (e.g., pulmonary or alveolar); external respiration.

x. volume of air in the lungs following a maximal expiration.

y. random movement of molecules from an area of high concentration to an area of low concentration.

Answers

Multiple Choice		True and False		Terms and Definitions	
1.	b	1.	False	1.	k
2.	a	2.	True	2.	o
3.	d	3.	True	3.	e
4.	d	4.	False	4.	l
5.	d	5.	True	5.	c
6.	a	6.	False	6.	g
7.	c	7.	False	7.	s
8.	a	8.	False	8.	n
9.	b	9.	True	9.	d
10.	b	10.	False	10.	f
11.	a	11.	True	11.	y
12.	b	12.	True	12.	m
13.	c	13.	False	13.	v
14.	d	14.	True	14.	j
15.	d	15.	False	15.	p
16.	d	16.	False	16.	a
17.	c	17.	True	17.	q
18.	a	18.	True	18.	x
19.	b	19.	False	19.	h
20.	a	20.	True	20.	b
				21.	t
				22.	u
				23.	w
				24.	i
				25.	r

Chapter 11: Acid-Base Balance During Exercise

Chapter Learning Objectives

After studying this chapter you should be able to do the following:

1. Define the terms *acid, base,* and *pH.*
2. Discuss the importance of acid-base regulation to exercise performance.
3. List the principal intracellular and extracellular buffers.
4. Explain the role of respiration in the regulation of acid-base status during exercise.
5. Outline acid-base regulation during exercise.
6. Discuss the principal ways that hydrogen ions are produced during exercise.

Multiple Choice

Instructions: After reading the question, and all possible answers, select the letter of choice that *BEST* answers the question. *Read all possible answers because some questions may have more than one correct answer.* The correct answers are provided at the end of this chapter.

1. Acidosis results from
    a. an accumulation of acids and/or a loss of bases.
    b. a decreased hydrogen ion concentration.
    c. hyperventilating.
    d. All of the above.

2. Exercise results in the production of large amounts of lactic acid which
    a. is produced by contracting skeletal muscle.
    b. ionizes and releases hydrogen ions.
    c. is an organic acid.
    d. All of the above.

3. The most common intracellular buffers are
    a. proteins and phosphate groups.
    b. weak acids.
    c. proteins, hemoglobin and bicarbonate.
    d. proteins, hemoglobin and phosphate groups.

4. Hemoglobin has approximately six times the buffering capacity of plasma proteins due to
    a. its high concentration.
    b. the ability of deoxygenated hemoglobin to buffer is greater than oxygenated hemoglobin.
    c. its ability to transport the plasma proteins.
    d. Both a and b are correct.

5. Ingestion of bicarbonate has been shown to
    a. improve performance in some types of exercise.
    b. improve performance in all types of exercise.
    c. increase blood bicarbonate concentration.
    d. Both a and c are correct.

6. The kidney is not an important regulator of acid-base balance during exercise because
    a. it can only decrease the rate of bicarbonate excretion.
    b. it can only increase the rate of bicarbonate excretion.
    c. it responds too slowly to be of major benefit.
    d. it is not capable of regulating hydrogen ion concentration.

7. The amount of lactic acid produced during exercise is dependent upon
   a. the exercise intensity.
   b. the muscle mass involved.
   c. the duration.
   d. All of the above.

8. Intracellular proteins are responsible for approximately
   a. 60% of the cells buffering capacity.
   b. 20-30% of the cells buffering capacity.
   c. 10-20% of the cells buffering capacity.
   d. None of the above.

9. The most important extracellular buffer is
   a. blood proteins.
   b. hemoglobin.
   c. phosphate groups.
   d. bicarbonate.

10. Respiratory compensation for metabolic alkalosis refers to
    a. the increase in the lactic acid production.
    b. the increase in ventilation resulting in a decrease in PCO_2.
    c. the decrease in ventilation resulting in an decrease in PCO_2.
    d. the decrease in ventilation resulting in an increase in PCO_2.

11. Intense exercise can cause blood pH to decline to
    a. 6.2.
    b. 6.8.
    c. 3.8.
    d. 5.2.

12. The Henderson-Hasselbach equation can be used to calculate
    a. the partial pressure of a gas.
    b. the pH of a solution by comparing the ratio of the concentration of the bicarbonate with the concentration of the base in solution.
    c. the pH of a solution by comparing the ratio of the concentration of the base with the concentration of the acid in solution.
    d. None of the above.

13. Buffers protect against pH change by
    a. removing hydrogen ions.
    b. releases hydrogen ions when pH increases.
    c. removing hydrogen ions when pH increases.
    d. None of the above.

14. Volatile acids include
    a. carbon dioxide and oxygen.
    b. carbon dioxide and carbonic acid.
    c. bicarbonate and hydrogen ions.
    d. sulfuric acid and phosphoric acid.

15. Respiratory compensation for metabolic acidosis causes a/an
    a. reduction in arterial PCO_2.
    b. decrease in arterial PCO_2.
    c. increase in blood bicarbonate.
    d. decrease in hydrogen ion production.

True and False

Instructions: Read each question carefully and determine if the statement is true or false. The correct answers to this exam are provided at the end of the chapter.

1. Bases that ionize completely are defined as strong bases.

2. An increase in the concentration of H^+ can be caused by an accumulation of bases.

3. CO_2 is termed a fixed acid as it needs to be eliminated by the lungs.

4. Intracellular phosphocreatine has been shown to be a useful buffer at the onset of exercise.

5. The bicarbonate buffer system is probably the most important buffer system in the body.

6. It is the partial pressure of oxygen in the blood that determines the concentration of carbonic acid.

7. When the amount of CO_2 in the blood increases the amount of H_2CO_3 decreases.

8. When the CO_2 content of the blood is lowered the pH of the blood decreases.

9. The decrease in muscle and blood pH during near maximal exercise is due to the production of lactic acid.

10. Evidence suggests that sodium bicarbonate ingestion can improve performance in long duration events.

11. Muscle bicarbonate contributes around 20-30% of the cell's buffering capacity.

12. At approximately 50-60% VO_2 max there is a decline in blood pH.

13. An increase in alveolar ventilation results in an increase in blood PCO_2.

14. A decrease in blood PCO_2 acts to reduce the acid load produced by exercise.

15. Failure to maintain acid-base homeostasis will impair metabolic pathways responsible for the production of ATP.

Matching Terms and Definitions

Instructions: Consider each term carefully and select the correct definition below. The correct answers are provided at the end of the chapter.

Terms
1. acidosis
2. acids
3. alkalosis
4. bases
5. buffers
6. hydrogen ion
7. ion
8. pH
9. respiratory compensation
10. strong acids
11. strong bases

Definitions

a. A free hydrogen ion in solution.

b. A measure of the acidity of a solution.

c. An abnormal increase in blood hydrogen ion concentration (i.e. arterial pH below 7.35).

d. A single atom or small molecule containing a net positive or negative charge due to an excess of either protons or electrons, respectively.

e. A base (alkaline substance) that completely ionizes when dissolved in water to generate OH^- and its cation.

f. A compound that ionizes in water to release hydroxyl ions (OH^-) or other ions that are capable of combining with hydrogen ions.

g. Resists pH change by removing hydrogen ions when the hydrogen ion concentration increases, and releasing hydrogen ions when the hydrogen ion concentration falls.

h. The buffering of excess H^+ in the blood by plasma bicarbonate (HCO_3^-), and the associated elevation in ventilation to exhale the resulting CO_2.

i. An abnormal increase in blood concentration of OH^- ions, resulting in a rise in arterial pH above 7.45.

j. A compound capable of giving up hydrogen ions into solution.

k. An acid that completely ionizes when dissolved in water to generate H^- and its anion.

Answers

Multiple Choice		True and False		Terms and Definitions	
1.	a	1.	True	1.	c
2.	d	2.	False	2.	j
3.	a	3.	False	3.	i
4.	a	4.	True	4.	f
5.	d	5.	True	5.	g
6.	c	6.	False	6.	a
7.	d	7.	False	7.	d
8.	a	8.	False	8.	b
9.	d	9.	True	9.	h
10.	b	10.	False	10.	k
11.	b	11.	True	11.	e
12.	c	12.	True		
13.	a	13.	False		
14.	b	14.	True		
15.	a	15.	True		

Chapter 12: Temperature Regulation

Chapter Learning Objectives

After studying this chapter you should be able to do the following:

1. Define the term *homeotherm*.
2. Present an overview of heat balance during exercise.
3. Discuss the concept of "core temperature."
4. List the principal means of involuntarily increasing heat production.
5. Define the four processes by which the body can lose heat during exercise.
6. Discuss the role of the hypothalamus as the body's thermostat.
7. Explain the thermal events that occur during exercise in both a cool/moderate and hot/humid environment.
8. List the physiological adaptations that occur during acclimatization to heat.
9. Describe the physiological responses to a cold environment.
10. Discuss the physiological changes that occur in response to cold acclimatization.

Multiple Choice

Instructions: After reading the question, and all possible answers, select the letter of choice that *BEST* answers the question. *Read all possible answers because some questions may have more than one correct answer.* The correct answers are provided at the end of this chapter.

1. If heat loss is less than heat production there will be a
   a. gain in body temperature.
   b. loss of body temperature.
   c. no change in body temperature.
   d. initial loss then a gain in body temperature.

2. During exercise, body temperature is regulated by making adjustments in
   a. the amount of heat produced.
   b. the resting metabolic rate.
   c. the amount of heat lost.
   d. biochemical heat production.

3. The temperature control center is in an area of the brain called the
   a. medulla.
   b. pons.
   c. pituitary.
   d. hypothalamus.

4. The amount of energy expended during exercise that appears as heat is approximately
   a. 20-25%.
   b. 40-45%.
   c. 55-60%.
   d. 75-80%.

5. A hormone released from the thyroid gland that is responsible for increasing the metabolic rate is/are
   a. epinephrine.
   b. thyroxine.
   c. norepinephrine.
   d. Both a and c are correct.

6. Radiative heat loss involves
   a. heat transfer to air molecules.
   b. heat transfer to water molecules.
   c. infrared rays.
   d. None of the above are correct.

7. Evaporation accounts for approximately _____ of the heat loss at rest
   a. 25%.
   b. 10%.
   c. 75%.
   d. 90%.

8. The least amount of evaporative cooling occurs on a
   a. hot/low humidity day.
   b. hot/high humidity day.
   c. cold/low humidity day.
   d. cold/high humidity day.

9. When air temperature is greater than skin temperature the only means of losing body heat during exercise is via
   a. radiation.
   b. conduction.
   c. convection.
   d. evaporation.

10. The vasomotor control center *is responsible* for the
    a. sweating response.
    b. detection of skin temperature.
    c. baroreceptor reflex.
    d. skin blood flow.

11. The rise in core temperature during exercise is most influenced by
    a. environmental temperature.
    b. relative humidity.
    c. exercise intensity.
    d. resting metabolic rate.

12. As the ambient temperature increases, the rate of convective and radiative heat loss
    a. decreases.
    b. increases.
    c. does not change.
    d. increases then decreases.

13. Heat acclimatization results in a _____ increase in plasma volume
    a. 10-12%.
    b. 4-6%.
    c. 20-22%.
    d. 30-32%.

14. Heat acclimatization is almost complete after
    a. 3-7 days.
    b. 7-14 days.
    c. 3-4 weeks.
    d. 1-2 months.

15. Cold acclimatization results in
    a. decrease in nonshivering thermogenesis.
    b. decreased peripheral circulation.
    c. improved ability to sleep in the cold.
    d. All of the above.

16. Exercise in a cold environment
    a. reduces an athlete's ability to lose heat.
    b. enhances an athlete's ability to lose heat.
    c. increases the chance of heat injury.
    d. Both a and c are correct.

17. During prolonged exercise in a moderate environment
    a. core temperature will increase gradually.
    b. core temperature will decrease gradually.
    c. core temperature will remain unchanged.
    d. core temperature will decrease then increase.

18. The organ that is responsible for reacting to increases in core temperature is the
    a. posterior hypothalamus.
    b. thyroid gland.
    c. anterior hypothalamus.
    d. Both b and c are correct.

19. Actions that are aimed at increasing heat loss are
    a. earlier commencement of sweating.
    b. increase in skin blood flow.
    c. cutaneous vasoconstriction.
    d. Both a and b are correct.

20. During 25 minutes of submaximal exercise in a cool environment which mechanism plays the least important role in heat loss?
    a. radiation
    b. conduction
    c. convection
    d. evaporation

True and False

Instructions: Read each question carefully and determine if the statement is true or false. The correct answers to this exam are provided at the end of the chapter.

1. Temperature homeostasis is maintained by an equal rate of body heat gain and heat loss.

2. Many exercise scientists believe that the only serious threat to health that exercise presents would be due to overheating.

3. One of the most common sites for core temperature measurement is the skin.

4. At rest, metabolic heat production is relatively large.

5. Involuntary heat production is the primary means of increasing heat production in the cold.

6. Evaporation occurs due to a vapor pressure gradient between the skin and the air.

7. At high environmental temperatures, relative humidity is the most important factor determining the rate of heat loss.

8. Under conditions of low humidity, cooling by convection is the most effective.

9. High sweat rates during exercise in a hot/high-humidity environment results in useless water loss.

10. There is a consistent decrease in evaporative heat loss with increments in exercise intensity.

11. There are marked differences in sweat rates and core temperatures during exercise in different environments.

12. At rest men are less heat tolerant than women.

13. Heat acclimatization results in a later onset of sweating.

14. People who are cold acclimatized begin shivering at lower skin temperatures.

15. Men tolerate mild cold exposure better than women.

16. During prolonged exercise in a moderate environment core temperature will increase gradually and reach a plateau.

17. During prolonged exercise in a hot/humid environment core does not reach a plateau.

18. Sweat losses of electrolytes are reduced after acclimatization due to an increased secretion of aldosterone.

19. Exercise training in sweat clothing in cool conditions will not promote heat acclimatization.

20. Cutaneous vasodilation will reduce heat loss.

Matching Terms and Definitions
Instructions: Consider each term carefully and select the correct definition below. The correct answers are provided at the end of the chapter.

Terms
1. anterior hypothalamus
2. conduction
3. convection
4. evaporation
5. homeotherms
6. hyperthermia
7. hypothermia
8. posterior hypothalamus
9. radiation

Definitions
a. Animals that maintain a fairly constant internal temperature.
b. A condition in which heat is lost from the body faster than it is produced.
c. The change of water from a liquid form to a vapor form.
d. Responsible for dealing with increases in body heat.
e. Process of energy exchange from the surface of one object to the surface of another not in direct contact.

f. Transfer of heat from warmer to cooler objects.
g. Responsible for the body's response to a decrease in temperature.
h. Transmission of heat from one object to another through the circulation of heated molecules.
i. An above-normal increase in body temperature.

Answers

Multiple Choice		True and False		Terms and Definitions	
1.	a	1.	True	1.	d
2.	c	2.	True	2.	f
3.	d	3.	False	3.	h
4.	d	4.	False	4.	c
5.	b	5.	True	5.	a
6.	c	6.	True	6.	i
7.	a	7.	True	7.	b
8.	b	8.	False	8.	g
9.	d	9.	True	9.	e
10.	d	10.	False		
11.	c	11.	True		
12.	a	12.	False		
13.	a	13.	False		
14.	b	14.	True		
15.	c	15.	False		
16.	b	16.	True		
17.	a	17.	True		
18.	c	18.	True		
19.	d	19.	False		
20.	a	20.	False		

Chapter 13: The Physiology of Training: Effect on VO$_2$ Max, Performance, Homeostasis and Strength

Chapter Learning Objectives

After studying this chapter you should be able to do the following:

1. Explain the basic principles of training: overload and specificity.
2. Contrast cross-sectional with longitudinal research studies.
3. Indicate the typical change in VO$_2$ max with endurance training programs, and the effect of the initial (pretraining) value on the magnitude of the increase.
4. State typical VO$_2$ max values for various patient, sedentary, active, and athletic populations.
5. State the formula for VO$_2$ max using heart rate, stroke volume, and the a-v O$_2$ difference; indicate which of the variables is most important in explaining the wide range of VO$_2$ max values in the population.
6. Discuss, using the variables identified in objective 5, how the increase in VO$_2$ max comes about for the sedentary subject who participates in an endurance training program.
7. Define preload, afterload, and contractility, and discuss the role of each in the increase in the maximal stroke volume that occurs with endurance training.
8. Describe the changes in muscle structure that are responsible for the increase in the maximal a-v O$_2$ difference with endurance training.
9. Describe the underlying causes of the decrease in VO$_2$ max that occurs with cessation of endurance training.
10. Describe how the capillary, myoglobin, and mitochondrial changes that occur in muscle as a result of an endurance training program are related to the following adaptations to submaximal exercise:
    a) a lower O$_2$ deficit
    b) an increased utilization of FFA and a sparing of blood glucose and muscle glycogen
    c) a reduction in lactate and H$^+$ formation
    d) an increase in lactate removal
11. Discuss how changes in "central command" and "peripheral feedback" following an endurance training program can lower the heart rate, ventilation, and catecholamine responses to a submaximal exercise bout.
12. Contrast the role of neural adaptations to that of hypertrophy in the increase in strength that occurs with resistance training.

Multiple Choice

Instructions: After reading the question, and all possible answers, select the letter of choice that *BEST* answers the question. *Read all possible answers because some questions may have more than one correct answer.* The correct answers are provided at the end of this chapter.

1. The typical variable(s) that constitute the overload in an endurance training program include
   a. intensity.
   b. duration.
   c. frequency.
   d. All of the above.

2. Individuals that begin endurance training programs with *high* VO_2 max values show improvements in VO_2 max in the range of _____ after two to three months.
   a. 2%-3%.
   b. 15%-20%.
   c. 25%-30%.
   d. 20%-25%.

3. Individuals that begin endurance training programs with *low* VO2 max values show improvements in VO2 max in the range of _____ after two to three months.
   a. 10%-20%.
   b. 20%-30%.
   c. 30%-50%.
   d. 50%-60%.

4. Which of the following VO_2 max values would be representative of a male cross country skier?
   a. 18 ml/kg/min.
   b. 50 ml/kg/min.
   c. 84 ml/kg/min.
   d. 67 ml/kg/min.

5. Which of the following VO_2 max values would be representative of individuals suffering from severe pulmonary disease?
   a. 5 ml/kg/min.
   b. 13 ml/kg/min.
   c. 25 ml/kg/min.
   d. None of the above.

6. Which of the following formulas could be used to calculate VO_2 max?
   a. HR max x SV max x (a-v O_2 difference) max
   b. HR x SV x (a-v O_2 difference)
   c. HR x SV x (a-v O_2 difference) max
   d. None of the above.

7. Cross sectional comparisons of groups differing in their level of habitual activity have shown that _____ is the variable that is the prime determinant of VO_2 max.
   a. number of mitochondria
   b. heart rate
   c. stroke volume
   d. a-v O_2 difference

8. Longitudinal studies have shown that training causes an increase in VO_2 max by
   a. increasing both stroke volume and the a-v O_2 difference.
   b. increasing stroke volume only.
   c. increasing the a-v O_2 difference only.
   d. decreasing the a-v O_2 difference.

9. Which of the following would cause an increase in stroke volume?
   a. an increase in end diastolic volume.
   b. an increase in myocardial contractility.
   c. a decrease in afterload.
   d. All of the above.

10. Which of the following statements is true of endurance trained muscle during maximal work?
    a. resistance to blood flow is increased
    b. resistance to blood flow is decreased
    c. resistance to blood flow does not change
    d. None of the above.

11. The increased capacity of the muscle to extract O_2 following an endurance training program is believed to be *primarily* due to
    a. the increase in capillary density.
    b. the increase in mitochondrial number.
    c. the increase in mitochondrial enzymes.
    d. Both b and c are correct.

12. During the initial 12 days of detraining the decrease in VO_2 max in highly trained individuals is *primarily* due to
    a. a decrease in both stroke volume and the a-v O_2 difference.
    b. a decrease in the a-v O_2 difference.
    c. a decrease in stroke volume.
    d. a decrease in heart rate maximum.

13. After an endurance training program oxidative phosphorylation is activated earlier at the onset of work and results in
    a. a faster rise in the oxygen uptake curve.
    b. a lower O_2 deficit.
    c. less lactate formation.
    d. All of the above.

14. After an endurance training program there is an increased utilization of fat, and sparing of carbohydrate. This is due to
    a. an increased reliance on glycolysis.
    b. an increased ability to transport FFA to the mitochondria.
    c. an increase in the fatty acid cycle enzymes.
    d. Both b and c are correct.

15. Endurance training shifts LDH toward the _____ isoform, making lactate and H^+ formation less likely and the uptake of pyruvate by the mitochondria more likely.
    a. M_4
    b. M_3H
    c. H_4
    d. M_2H_2

16. Endurance training causes an increase in the capillary density of the working muscles. This results in
    a. a decrease in the distance from capillary to mitochondria.
    b. a slower red blood cell transit time through the muscle.
    c. decreased oxygen extraction from each liter of blood.
    d. Both a and b are correct.

17. With the increase in mitochondria number following endurance training, local factors (H^+, adenosine compounds etc.) do not change as much. This leads to
    a. increased chemoreceptor input to the cardiorespiratory centers.
    b. less local stimulation of blood flow.
    c. increased local stimulation of blood flow.
    d. increased feedback from the muscle.

18. Increases in strength due to short-term training are the result of
    a. hypertrophy.
    b. neural adaptations.
    c. neural adaptations, hypertrophy, and hyperplasia.
    d. hyperplasia.

19. The decreases in VO_2 max with cessation of exercise are primarily due to a
    a. decrease in maximal stroke volume.
    b. decrease in oxygen extraction.
    c. decrease in myoglobin concentration.
    d. Both a and b are correct.

20. The relationship between varying amounts of exercise and the risk of infection is
    a. linear.
    b. s shaped.
    c. j shaped.
    d. exponential.

True and False

Instructions: Read each question carefully and determine if the statement is true or false. The correct answers to this exam are provided at the end of the chapter.

1. In cross-sectional studies the investigator examines different groups and analyses the differences.

2. VO_2 max can be less than 20 ml/kg/min. in patients with severe pulmonary disease and more than 80 ml/kg/min. in world class distance runners and cross-country skiers.

3. An increase in plasma volume can cause an increased stroke volume.

4. If the heart contracts with the same force while the peripheral resistance increases, a greater stroke volume will occur.

5. Type I muscle fibers develop more tension than type II fibers.

6. The increase in maximal stroke volume after endurance training is due to both a decrease in preload and an increase in afterload.

7. Between days 21 and 84 of detraining the decrease in VO_2 max is due to the decrease in the a-v O_2 difference.

8. Muscle cells with few mitochondria need only a low ADP concentration to stimulate the mitochondria to consume oxygen at a given rate.

9. After endurance training there is an increased reliance on anaerobic glycolysis to provide ATP at the onset of exercise.

10. Plasma FFA provide 90% of the fat oxidized by muscle during exercise.

11. The increase in capillary density at the muscle allows for a slower muscle capillary blood flow during exercise and an increased surface area for the diffusion of FFA into the muscle.

12. Carbohydrates are transported from the cytoplasm to the mitochondria by carnitine transferase, an enzyme associated with the mitochondrial membrane.

13. Low citrate levels inhibit PFK activity in the cytoplasm and therefore reduces carbohydrate metabolism.

14. The increase in mitochondria number after endurance training decreases the chance that pyruvate will be taken up by the mitochondria for oxidation in the Krebs cycle.

15. Heart rate, ventilation, and plasma catecholamine responses to prolonged submaximal exercise are determined by the training state of the specific muscle groups engaged in the exercise.

16. Mitochondrial oxidative capacity undergoes rapid changes at the onset of an exercise training program.

17. A muscle fiber's oxidative capacity will improve even if the fiber is not recruited during exercise.

18. Strenuous exercise is needed to change low oxidative (type IIb) fibers.

19. Excessive amounts of exercise has been shown to increase the risk of infection.

20. The loss of muscle mass with aging occurs in only type IIb fibers.

Matching Terms and Definitions

Instructions: Consider each term carefully and select the correct definition below. The correct answers are provided at the end of the chapter.

Terms
1. bradycardia
2. ejection fraction
3. overload
4. reversibility
5. specificity

Definitions
a. A principle of training describing the need to increase the load (intensity) of exercise at a level beyond which is presently accustomed in order for a training effect to occur.
b. The training effect is specific to the muscle fibers involved in the exercise.
c. A resting heart rate less than sixty beats per minute.
d. The proportion of end diastolic volume that is ejected during a ventricular contraction.
e. The training effect is lost when the overload or training stimulus is removed.

Answers

Multiple Choice	True and False	Terms and Definitions
1. d	1. True	1. c
2. a	2. True	2. d
3. c	3. True	3. a
4. c	4. False	4. e
5. b	5. True	5. b
6. a	6. False	
7. c	7. True	
8. a	8. False	
9. d	9. False	
10. c	10. False	
11. a	11. True	
12. c	12. False	
13. d	13. False	
14. d	14. False	
15. c	15. True	
16. d	16. True	
17. b	17. False	
18. b	18. True	
19. d	19. True	
20. c	20. False	

Chapter 14: Patterns in Health and Disease

Chapter Learning Objectives

After studying this chapter you should be able to do the following:

1. Define or describe the science of epidemiology.
2. Contrast infectious with degenerative diseases as causes of death.
3. Identify the three major categories of risk factors and examples of specific risk factors in each.
4. Compare the epidemiologic triad with the web of causation as models to study infectious and degenerative diseases respectively.
5. Describe the difference between primary and secondary risk factors for coronary heart disease (CHD).
6. Describe the steps an epidemiologist must follow to show that a risk factor is causally connected to a disease.
7. Describe the hypothesis linking resistance to insulin as a cause of hypertension.

Multiple Choice

Instructions: After reading the question, and all possible answers, select the letter of choice that *BEST* answers the question. *Read all possible answers because some questions may have more than one correct answer.* The correct answers are provided at the end of this chapter.

1. The epidemiologic triad shows the interaction of
   a. environment, host and behavior.
   b. genetics environment and behavior.
   c. environment, host and agent.
   d. None of the above.

2. An epidemiological model that attempts to establish cause by showing the interaction of risk factors is
   a. web of epidemiological triad
   b. web of epidemiology
   c. web of causation
   d. none of the above

3. Which of the following is a degenerative disease ?
   a. influenza.
   b. pneumonia.
   c. cardiovascular disease.
   d. None of the above.

4. Which of the following is an infectious disease ?
   a. tuberculosis.
   b. cancer.
   c. cardiovascular disease.
   d. None of the above.

5. The major cause of death in the United States in 1991 was
   a. tuberculosis.
   b. accidents.
   c. cardiovascular disease.
   d. cancer.

6. Our understanding of the risks associated with atherosclerotic disease is based more on
   a. genetic research.
   b. environmental research.
   c. animal research.
   d. epidemiological research.

7. The Framingham study found that the risk factor/s that contributed to heart disease were
   a. smoking.
   b. hypertension..
   c. high cholesterol.
   d. All of the above.

8. Atherosclerosis is the term used to describe
   a. the hardening of the arteries.
   b. narrowing of the coronary arteries.
   c. high blood pressure.
   d. the onset of a heart attack.

9. Which of the following is a primary risk factor for coronary heart disease?
   a. high blood pressure.
   b. diabetes.
   c. obesity.
   d. stress.

10. Which of the following is a secondary or contributing risk factor for coronary heart disease?
    a. high serum cholesterol.
    b. cigarette smoking.
    c. diabetes.
    d. physical inactivity.

11. The decrease in the death rate from heart disease and stroke since 1970 is related to
    a. the decline in cigarette smoking.
    b. increased monitoring of blood pressure.
    c. increased awareness of the role of blood cholesterol and dietary fat.
    d. All of the above.

12. The nutrition objectives for coronary heart disease risk reduction indicate a need to
    a. decrease fat intake.
    b. decrease salt intake.
    c. increase intake of complex carbohydrates.
    d. All of the above.

13. The deadly quartet model describes potential causative connections between and among
    a. obesity, hypertension, insulin resistance and dyslipidemia.
    b. heart disease, obesity, hypertension and tuberculosis.
    c. hypertension, tuberculosis, heart disease and obesity.
    d. None of the above.

14. Insulin resistance is located primarily in
    a. type I fibers.
    b. type IIa fibers.
    c. all type II fibers.
    d. type Ia fibers.

15. Mean arterial blood pressure is higher in subjects with a high percentage of
    a. type I fibers.
    b. type IIa fibers.
    c. all type II fibers.
    d. type Ia fibers.

16. To facilitate the process of determining cause, epidemiologists might apply the following guideline/s
    a. temporal disassociation.
    b. factuality.
    c. consistency.
    d. all of the above.

True and False

Instructions: Read each question carefully and determine if the statement is true or false. The correct answers to this exam are provided at the end of the chapter.

1. Epidemiology is where you hypothesize the outcome of a disease.

2. The effectiveness of the treatment of a disease can only be evaluated if the natural history of the disease in the absence of a treatment is known.

3. Physical inactivity is an independent risk factor for coronary heart disease.

4. During the course of the twentieth century the major causes of death in the United States have shifted from degenerative diseases to infectious diseases.

5. It is generally agreed that health means more than the simple absence of disease.

6. Degenerative diseases have more complex causes than infectious diseases and therefore are not preventable.

7. The ratio of total cholesterol to HDL-C is viewed as a better index of risk than total cholesterol alone.

8. A high fat diet may not be listed as a risk factor for CHD because its effect is already considered in the factors of high cholesterol and obesity.

9. A primary risk factor is one that increases risk when another primary risk factor is present.

10. A secondary risk factor is one that exerts an independent effect on a disease.

11. Exercise can both directly and indirectly decrease the risk of coronary heart disease.

12. Insulin resistance is greater in type II fibers due to their limited capillary supply.

13. Around 50 million Americans have hypertension.

14. Insulin resistance is characterized by an increased ability to take up glucose.

15. Increased insulin secretion can lead to a decreased blood pressure.

Matching Terms and Definitions

Instructions: Consider each term carefully and select the correct definition. The correct answers are provided at the end of the chapter.

Terms
1. atherosclerosis
2. degenerative diseases
3. epidemiologic triad
4. epidemiology
5. infectious diseases
6. primary risk factor
7. secondary risk factor
8. web of causation

Definitions
a. A sign (e.g., high blood pressure) or a behavior (e.g., cigarette smoking) that is directly related to the appearance of certain diseases independent of other risk factors.
b. Diseases not due to infection, which result in a progressive decline in some bodily function.
c. The gradual narrowing of the coronary arteries due to a build up of fatty substances in the inner lining of the artery.
d. A characteristic or behavior that increases the risk of coronary heart disease when primary risk factors are present.
e. Diseases due to the presence of pathogenic microorganisms in the body (e.g., viruses, bacteria, fungi, and protozoa).
f. The study of the distribution and determinants of health related states.
g. Epidemiological model that shows the connections between the environment, agent and host that cause disease.
h. Epidemiological model that shows the complex interactions of risk factors associated with a disease.

Answers

Multiple Choice	True and False	Terms and Definitions
1. b	1. False	1. c
2. c	2. True	2. b
3. c	3. True	3. g
4. a	4. False	4. f
5. c	5. True	5. e
6. d	6. False	3. a
7. d	7. True	4. d
8. b	8. True	5. h
9. a	9. False	
10. c	10. False	
11. d	11. True	
12. d	12. True	
13. a	13. True	
14. c	14. False	
15. c	15. False	
16. c		

Chapter 15: Work Tests to Evaluate Cardiorespiratory Fitness

Chapter Learning Objectives

After studying this chapter you should be able to do the following:

1. Identify the sequence of steps in the procedures for evaluating cardiorespiratory fitness (CRF).
2. Describe one maximal and one submaximal field test used to evaluate CRF.
3. Explain the rationale underlying the use of distance runs as estimates of CRF.
4. Identify the common measures taken during a graded exercise test (GXT).
5. Describe changes in the ECG that may take place during a GXT of subjects with ischemic heart disease.
6. List three criteria for having achieved VO_2 max.
7. Estimate VO_2 max from the last stage of a GXT and list the concerns about the protocol that may affect that estimate.
8. Estimate VO_2 max by extrapolating a HR/VO_2 relationship to the person's age-adjusted maximal HR.
9. Describe the problems with the assumptions made in the extrapolation procedure used in objective 9, and name the environmental and subject variables that must be controlled to improve such estimates.
10. Identify the criteria used to terminate the GXT.
11. Explain why there are so many different GXT protocols and why the rate of progression through the test is of concern.
12. Describe a procedure used to set the initial work rate and the rate of progression on a cycle ergometer test.
13. Estimate VO_2 max with the Astrand and Rhyming nomogram, given a data set for the cycle ergometer or step.

Multiple Choice

Instructions: After reading the question, and all possible answers, select the letter of choice that *BEST* answers the question. *Read all possible answers because some questions may have more than one correct answer.* The correct answers are provided at the end of this chapter.

1. The type of graded exercise test (GXT) used depends on
   a. the fitness of the person being tested.
   b. the purpose of the test.
   c. facilities, equipment, and personnel available.
   d. All of the above.

2. Identify the sequence of steps in the procedures for evaluating cardiorespiratory function (CRF)
   a. informed consent, health history, resting physiological measures, GXT.
   b. informed consent, resting physiological measures, GXT, health history.
   c. health history, GXT, informed consent, resting physiological measures.
   d. None of the above.

3. Individuals who have some form of coronary, pulmonary, or metabolic disease
   a. may take a GXT as long as it is within one mile from a hospital.
   b. must be referred to a physician before taking a GXT.
   c. do not need to be referred to a physician before taking a GXT.
   d. should not take a GXT.

4. Which of the following is/are true of a diagnostic graded exercise test (GXT)?
   a. heart rate and blood pressure are not taken prior to the test.
   b. a resting ECG is always taken prior to the test.
   c. a blood sample is always taken.
   d. Both a and b are correct.

5. Which of the following abnormal resting values would require medical consultation prior to taking the GXT?
   a. heart rate
   b. blood pressure
   c. ECG
   d. All of the above.

6. Which of the following cardiorespiratory fitness (CRF) tests is a maximal test that is not "graded" and does not require physiological measurements to be made?
   a. Cooper's 12-minute run.
   b. VO_2 max test on the treadmill.
   c. AAHPERD's 1-mile run.
   d. Both a and c are correct.

7. Which of the following is an advantage of using a field test for estimating CRF?
   a. it is easy to monitor physiological responses.
   b. the test is graded.
   c. they have a moderately high correlation with VO_2 max.
   d. All of the above.

8. During the walk test which physiological parameter is measured?
   a. blood pressure.
   b. heart rate.
   c. ECG.
   d. VO_2 max.

9. An estimate of the work (and O_2 demand) of the heart is
   a. the product of heart rate and mean blood pressure.
   b. the product of the heart rate and the systolic blood pressure.
   c. the product of the heart rate and the diastolic blood pressure.
   d. None of the above.

10. Which of the following is an ECG sign associated with myocardial ischemia?
    a. ST segment depression
    b. PQ segment depression
    c. PT segment depression
    d. QR segment depression

11. Which of the following would indicate that VO_2 max had been achieved during a GXT?
    a. a leveling off of the VO_2 even though a higher work rate is achieved
    b. a post exercise blood lactate level of <5 mmoles/liter
    c. R exceeding 8.5
    d. All of the above.

12. The highest value for VO_2 max is usually measured with
    a. a walking test up a grade on a treadmill.
    b. a running test up a grade on a treadmill.
    c. a cycle ergometer.
    d. a running test with no grade on a treadmill.

13. If the increments in a GXT are too short for an individual to achieve a steady state, the following will result
    a. VO_2 max will be underestimated.
    b. VO_2 max will be overestimated.
    c. prediction of VO_2 max will not be affected.
    d. peak VO_2 will be reached rather than VO_2 max.

14. A common measurement made at each stage of the GXT is Borg's Rating of Perceived Exertion (RPE). The RPE scores are
    a. poor indicators of subjective effort.
    b. provide a quantitative way to track a person's progress.
    c. provide an accurate VO_2 max value.
    d. Both a and b are correct.

15. Which of the following would require the GXT to be terminated
    a. subject request to stop
    b. failure of the monitoring system
    c. dyspnea
    d. All of the above

True and False

Instructions: Read each question carefully and determine if the statement is true or false. The correct answers are provided at the end of the chapter.

1. The first step in the evaluation of CRF is to screen the subject.

2. PAR-Q is a form used to determine if a person needs a consultation with a physician before taking a GXT.

3. The basis for the field tests is the linear relationship that exists between VO_2 (ml/kg/min.) and running speed.

4. The formulas used for estimating VO_2 max on a 12-minute run are useful for prepubescent children since their economy of running is similar to that of an adult.

5. VO_2 peak is the term used to describe the highest VO_2 achieved on walk, cycle, or arm ergometer protocols.

6. Estimation of VO_2 max from heart rate values during a series of submaximal work rates is a simple and commonly used procedure with no known problems.

7. The GXT protocols can be either submaximal or maximal, depending on the end points used to stop the test.

8. GXT protocols should not vary in terms of the initial work rate, the increment in work rate between stages, and the duration of each stage.

9. The Standard Balke protocol is suitable for most average sedentary adults.

10. A GXT for young active subjects would have an initial work rate of approximately 6 METS with increments of 2-3 METS per stage.

11. The heart rate response during a GXT is usually linear between 110 beats per minute and 85% of maximal heart rate.

12. For a small person the relative VO_2 at any work rate on a cycle ergometer is higher than for a big person.

13. VO_2 max can be estimated with the extrapolation procedure using the treadmill, cycle ergometer, or step.

14. For the extrapolation procedure to estimate VO_2 max to be accurate the environmental conditions must be controlled.

15. The step test protocol is not used the same way to estimate VO_2 max.

Matching Terms and Definitions

Instructions: Consider each term carefully and select the correct definition below. The correct answers are provided at the end of the chapter.

Terms
1. angina pectoris
2. arrhythmias
3. conduction disturbances
4. double product
5. dyspnea
6. field test
7. myocardial ischemia
8. ST segment depression

Definitions
a. A condition in which the myocardium experiences inadequate blood flow.
b. A test of physical performance performed in the field (outside the laboratory).
c. Shortness of breath or labored breathing.
d. Abnormal electrical activity in the heart.
e. Refers to a slowing or blockage of the wave of depolarization in the heart.
f. Chest pain due to a lack of blood flow to the myocardium.
g. The product of heart rate and systolic blood pressure.
h. An electrocardiographic change reflecting an ischemia in the heart muscle.

Answers

Multiple Choice	True and False	Terms and Definitions
1. d	1. True	1. f
2. a	2. True	2. d
3. b	3. True	3. e
4. b	4. False	4. g
5. d	5. True	5. c
6. d	6. False	6. b
7. c	7. True	7. a
8. b	8. False	8. h
9. b	9. True	
10. a	10. True	
11. a	11. True	
12. b	12. True	
13. b	13. True	
14. b	14. True	
15. d	15. True	

Chapter 16: Exercise Prescriptions for Health and Fitness

Chapter Learning Objectives

After studying this chapter you should be able to do the following:

1. Characterize physical inactivity as a coronary heart disease risk factor comparable to smoking, hypertension, and high serum cholesterol.
2. Contrast "exercise" with "physical activity"; explain how both relate to a lower risk of CHD and improvement in cardiorespiratory fitness (CRF).
3. Describe the "Exercise Lite" program recommended by the American College of Sports Medicine and the Centers for Disease Control and Prevention to improve the health status of U.S. adults.
4. Explain what "screening" and "progression" mean for a person wishing to initiate an exercise program.
5. Identify the optimal frequency, intensity, and duration of activity associated with improvements in CRF; why is more not necessarily better than less?
6. Calculate a target heart rate range by either the heart rate range or percent of maximal HR methods.
7. Explain why the appropriate sequence of physical activity for sedentary persons is walk ---> walk/jog ---> jog ---> games.
8. Explain how the target heart rate (THR) helps adjust exercise intensity in times of high heat, humidity, or while at altitude.

Multiple Choice

Instructions: After reading the question, and all possible answers, select the letter of choice that *BEST* answers the question. *Read all possible answers because some questions may have more than one correct answer.* The correct answers are provided at the end of this chapter.

1. The exercise dose is usually characterized by the
    a. intensity, frequency and duration.
    b. type of activity.
    c. response.
    d. Both a and b are correct.

2. Every U.S. adult should accumulate _____ minutes or more of moderate intensity physical activity on most days of the week
    a. 10.
    b. 30.
    c. 60.
    d. 90.

3. The Harvard Alumni Health Study showed that death from all causes is most linked to
    a. vigorous activity.
    b. non-vigorous activity.
    c. intermediate activity.
    d. None of the above.

4. The greatest health benefits appear when a formerly sedentary person becomes moderately active, that is, expending about _____ kcal at least every other day
    a. 200-300.
    b. 50-100.
    c. 75-150..
    d. 500-600..

5. The risk of cardiac arrest in vigorously active men is only _____ of the risk in sedentary men.
   a. 20%.
   b. 30%.
   c. 40%.
   d. 50%.

6. What type of activity is recommended early in a health-related exercise program for previously sedentary individuals?
   a. slow jogging.
   b. slow to moderate walking.
   c. brisk walking.
   d. fast jogging.

7. At the end of an activity session a cool-down period of slow walking and stretching for about five minutes is recommended to
   a. return heart rate toward normal.
   b. reduce the chance of a hypotensive episode.
   c. return blood pressure toward normal.
   d. All of the above.

8. How many exercise sessions are recommended each week in order to improve cardiorespiratory fitness?
   a. 2-3.
   b. 3-5.
   c. 5-7.
   d. 7.

9. How many minutes are recommended for each exercise session in order to improve cardiorespiratory fitness?
   a. 20-60
   b. 10-20
   c. 60-100
   d. None of the above.

10. What intensity (i.e. % of VO_2 max) does an individual need to exercise at in order to improve cardiorespiratory fitness?
    a. 20-30%
    b. 50-85%
    c. 40-50%
    d. Any of the above.

11. Exercise perceived as "somewhat hard," 12-14 on the original RPE scale approximates _____ of maximal heart rate
    a. 30-40%
    b. 40-50%
    c. 50-70%
    d. 70-85%

12. Which of the following is *not true* of the RPE scale?
    a. it is closely linked to the % VO_2 max
    b. it is closely linked to the lactate threshold
    c. it is dependent on the mode of exercise
    d. it has a high test reliability

13. The net energy cost of jogging
    a. is about twice that of walking for the same time period.
    b. is equal to that of walking for the same time period.
    c. requires a greater cardiovascular response than walking.
    d. Both a and c are correct.

14. As a participant adapts to jogging, the heart rate response for any jogging speed will
    a. increase.
    b. decrease.
    c. stay the same.
    d. decrease then increase.

15. In the latest position stand by the American College of Sports Medicine what was added?
    a. resistance training.
    b. endurance training.
    c. games and sports.
    d. jogging.

True and False

Instructions: Read each question carefully and determine if the statement is true or false. The correct answers are provided at the end of the chapter.

1. The American Heart Association has recognized physical inactivity as a primary risk factor for coronary heart disease.

2. Approximately 200-300 kcal will be expended when walking for about four miles at a moderate pace, or jogging about two miles.

3. A high VO_2 max has not been shown to be associated with a lower death rate.

4. The cardiorespiratory fitness training effect is dependent on the proper frequency, duration, and intensity of the exercise sessions.

5. Gains in cardiorespiratory fitness and weight loss can be achieved with a two day per week exercise program.

6. Once the minimal threshold of intensity is achieved total work accomplished per session seems to be the most important variable associated with improvements in cardiorespiratory fitness.

7. Engaging in strenuous exercise (75% VO_2 max) beyond 30 minutes increases the risk of orthopedic problems.

8. The Karvonen method of calculating the target heart rate range is a direct method.

9. Resistance training for the development of strength should be performed at least twice a week.

10. For strength gains to occur it is recommended that resistance exercises requiring a full range of motion at an intensity that would cause fatigue in 15-20 repetitions be performed.

11. As the heat and humidity increase, there is an increased need to circulate additional blood to the skin to dissipate the heat.

12. The target heart rate can act as a guide to adjust exercise intensity even in adverse environmental conditions.

13. A decrease in exercise intensity will not counter the effects of an adverse environment.

14. The intensity threshold for a training effect is higher for a fit individual compared to a sedentary person.

15. Strenuous exercise increases the risk of a heart attack during the activity.

Matching Terms and Definitions

Instructions: Consider each term carefully and select the correct definition below. The correct answers are provided at the end of the chapter.

Terms
1. dose
2. effect
3. exercise
4. physical activity
5. physical fitness
6. target heart rate (THR) range

Definitions
a. 70-85% HR max.
b. A broad term describing healthful levels of cardiovascular function, strength, and flexibility.
c. Characterizes all types of human movement; associated with living, work, play, and exercise.
d. A subclass of physical activity.
e. Desired response.
f. The quantity prescribed.

Answers

Multiple Choice	True and False	Terms and Definitions
1. d	1. True	1. f
2. b	2. True	2. e
3. a	3. False	3. d
4. a	4. True	4. c
5. c	5. False	5. b
6. b	6. True	6. a
7. d	7. False	7. b
8. b	8. False	8. a
9. a	9. True	
10. b	10. False	
11. d	11. True	
12. c	12. False	
13. d	13. False	
14. b	14. False	
15. a	15. True	

Chapter 17: Exercise for Special Populations

Chapter Learning Objectives

After studying this chapter you should be able to do the following:

1. Describe the difference between Type I and Type II diabetes.
2. Contrast how a diabetic responds to exercise when blood glucose is "in control", compared to when it is not.
3. Explain why exercise may complicate the life of a Type I diabetic, while being a recommended and primary part of a Type II diabetic's life-style.
4. Describe the changes in diet and insulin that might be made prior to a diabetic undertaking an exercise program.
5. Describe the sequence of events leading to an asthma attack, and how cromolyn sodium and β-adrenergic agonists act to prevent and/or relieve an attack.
6. Describe the cause of exercise-induced asthma, and how one may deal with this problem.
7. Contrast chronic obstructive pulmonary disease (COPD) with asthma in terms of causes, prognosis, and the role of rehabilitation programs in a return to "normal" function.
8. Identify the types of patient populations that one might see in a cardiac rehabilitation program, and the types of medications that these individuals may be taking.
9. Contrast the type of exercise test used for cardiac populations with the test used for the apparently healthy population.
10. Describe the physiological changes in the elderly that result from an endurance-training program.
11. Describe the guidelines for exercise programs for pregnant women.

Multiple Choice

Instructions: After reading the question, and all possible answers, select the letter of choice that *BEST* answers the question. *Read all possible answers because some questions may have more than one correct answer.* The correct answers are provided at the end of this chapter.

1. Which type of diabetes mellitus is caused by lack of insulin and is associated with viral (flulike) infections?
   a. Type I
   b. Type Ia
   c. Type II
   d. Type IIb

2. Which of the following is a warning sign for Type I diabetes?
   a. infrequent urination
   b. loss of appetite
   c. weakness and fatigue
   d. weight gain

3. Which form of diabetes is primarily linked to obesity?
   a. Type I
   b. Type II
   c. Type III
   d. All of the above

4. The primary treatment of Type II diabetes includes
   a. injecting insulin
   b. diet
   c. exercise
   d. Both b and c are correct.

5. If an insulin-dependent diabetic starts exercise with too much insulin, this may cause
   a. a dangerous hyperglycemic response.
   b. a dangerous hypoglycemic response.
   c. an increased rate of glucose release from the liver.
   d. a decreased rate of plasma glucose use by the muscle.

6. Hypoglycemia can lead to
   a. insulin shock.
   b. diabetic coma.
   c. ketosis.
   d. Any of the above.

7. An asthma attack is the result of an orderly sequence of events that can be initiated by a wide variety of factors. Which of the following is the initial event in this sequence?
   a. release of chemical mediators such as histamine
   b. increase in smooth muscle contraction
   c. increasing Ca^{++} influx into the mast cell
   d. inflammation response (swelling of tissue)

8. How does cromolyn sodium function to prevent an asthma attack?
   a. increases the activity of cyclic AMP
   b. inhibits phosphodiesterase
   c. inhibits the chemical mediator release from the mast cell
   d. acts as a beta receptor antagonist

9. Which of the following has been identified as a cause of exercise induced asthma (EIA)?
   a. cold air
   b. hypocapnia
   c. respiratory alkalosis
   d. All of the above.

10. Which of the following activities has the greatest probability of causing an exercise-induced bronchospasm?
    a. walking
    b. running
    c. cycling
    d. swimming

11. Which of the following is a common test used to classify COPD patients?
    a. FEV_1
    b. minimum exercise ventilation
    c. GXT to evaluate VO_2 max
    d. Both a and c are correct.

12. Heart damage (loss of ventricular muscle) due to prolonged occlusion of one or more of the coronary arteries is also known as
    a. coronary angioplasty.
    b. angina pectoris.
    c. coronary hypertrophy.
    d. myocardial infarction.

13. Type I osteoporosis is related to which of the following fractures?
    a. vertebral and distal radius
    b. hip
    c. pelvic
    d. distal humerus

14. Which of the following is an absolute contraindication for aerobic exercise during pregnancy?
    a. a history of premature labor
    b. multiple pregnancy
    c. anemia
    d. obesity

15. Maximal aerobic power decreases in the average population after the age of twenty at a rate of around
    a. 1% per year.
    b. 5% per year.
    c. 10% per year.
    d. 0.1% per year.

True and False

Instructions: Read each question carefully and determine if the statement is true or false. The correct answers are provided at the end of this chapter.

1. "Control" means that blood glucose concentration is close to normal.

2. When an insulin dependent diabetic does not inject an adequate amount of insulin before exercise hypoglycemia results.

3. If an insulin-dependent diabetic starts exercise with too much insulin, the rate at which plasma glucose is used by muscle is accelerated.

4. Type I diabetics represent about 90% of the whole population of diabetics.

5. Non insulin-dependent diabetics do not experience the same fluctuations in blood glucose during exercise as do the Type I diabetics.

6. It is believed that dust, chemicals, antibodies, and exercise initiate the asthma attack by increasing Ca^{++} influx into the mast cell.

7. A patient developing COPD still has the ability to perform normal activities without experiencing dyspnea.

8. Those with mild hypertension represent most of the morbidity and mortality associated with hypertension.

9. A blood pressure reading of 165/110 would be considered normal for a healthy adult.

10. There are no classes of CHD patients for whom exercise or exercise testing is inappropriate.

11. Exercise programs bring about large changes for CHD patients.

12. The guidelines for exercise training programs for the elderly are similar to those who are younger.

13. The effort required to bring about the training effect is more difficult in older individuals.

14. Endurance exercise can be done during pregnancy without complications to the mother or fetus.

15. Exercise training is still not considered a part of the therapy used with CHD patients.

Matching Terms and Definitions

Instructions: Consider each term carefully and select the correct definition below. The correct answers are provided at the end of the chapter.

Terms
1. beta receptor agonist
2. coronary artery bypass graft surgery (CABGS)
3. cromolyn sodium
4. diabetic coma
5. immunotherapy
6. insulin shock
7. ketosis
8. mast cell
9. myocardial infarction
10. nitroglycerin
11. percutaneous transluminal coronary angioplasty
12. theophylline

Definitions
a. Condition brought on by too much insulin, which causes an immediate hypoglycemia.
b. Connective tissue cell that releases histamine and other chemicals in response to certain stimuli.
c. A molecule that is capable of binding to and activating a beta receptor.
d. The replacement of a blocked coronary artery with another vessel to permit blood flow to the myocardium.
e. A drug used to stabilized the membranes of mast cells and prevent an asthma attack.
f. Death of a portion of heart tissue.
g. Unconscious state induced by a lack of insulin.
h. Procedure in which the body is exposed to substances to elicit an immune response in order to offer better protection upon subsequent exposure.
i. A balloon-tipped catheter is inserted into a blocked coronary artery and plaque is pushed back to artery wall to open the blood vessel.
j. Drug used to reduce chest pain due to lack of blood flow to the myocardium.
k. Acidosis of the blood caused by the production of ketone bodies when fatty acid mobilization is increased.
l. A drug used as a smooth muscle relaxant in the treatment of asthma.

Answers

Multiple Choice	True and False	Terms and Definitions
1. a	1. True	1. c
2. c	2. False	2. d
3. b	3. True	3. e
4. d	4. False	4. g
5. b	5. True	5. h
6. a	6. True	6. a
7. c	7. False	7. k
8. c	8. True	8. b
9. d	9. False	9. f
10. b	10. False	10. j
11. d	11. True	11. i
12. d	12. True	12. l
13. a	13. False	
14. b	14. True	
15. a	15. False	

Chapter 18: Body Composition and Nutrition for Health

Chapter Learning Objectives

After studying this chapter you should be able to do the following:

1. Identify the U.S. Dietary Goals relative to a) carbohydrates and fats as a percent of energy intake, b) salt and cholesterol, and c) saturated and unsaturated fats.
2. Contrast the Dietary Goals with the Dietary Guidelines.
3. Describe what is meant by the term *Recommended Dietary Allowance* (RDA), and how the RDA relates to the *Daily Value* (DV) used in food labeling.
4. List the classes of nutrients.
5. Identify the fat-and water-soluble vitamins, describe what toxicity is, and which class of vitamins is more likely to cause this problem.
6. Contrast major minerals with trace minerals, and describe the role of calcium, iron, and sodium in health and disease.
7. Identify the primary role of carbohydrates, the two major classes, and the recommended changes in the American diet to improve health status.
8. Identify the primary role of fat, and the recommended changes in the American diet to improve health status.
9. List the food groups and major nutrients represented in the Food Guide Pyramid.
10. Describe the Exchange System of planning diets, and how it differs from the Food Guide Pyramid.
11. Describe the limitation of the height/weight table in determining body composition.
12. Provide a brief description of the following methods of measuring body composition: isotope dilution, photon absorptiometry, potassium-40, hydrostatic (underwater weighing), dual energy x-ray absorptiometry, near infrared interactance, radiography, ultrasound, nuclear magnetic resonance, total body electrical conductivity, bioelectrical impedance analysis and skinfold thickness.
13. Describe the two-component system of body composition and the assumptions made about the density values for the fat-free mass and the fat mass.
14. Explain the principle underlying the measurement of whole body density with underwater weighing, and why one must correct for residual volume.
15. Explain why there is an error of $\pm 2.0\%$ in the calculation of percent body fat with the underwater weighing technique.
16. Explain how a sum of skinfolds can be "converted" to a percent body fatness value.
17. List the recommended percent body fatness values for health and fitness for males and females, and explain the concern for both high and low values.
18. Discuss the reasons why the average weight at any height (fatness) has increased while deaths from cardiovascular diseases have decreased.
19. Distinguish between obesity due to hyperplasia of fat cells and that due to hypertrophy of fat cells.
20. Describe the roles of genetics and environment in the appearance of obesity.
21. Explain the set point theory of obesity, and give an example of a physiological and behavioral control system.
22. Describe the pattern of change in body weight and caloric intake over the adult years.
23. Discuss the changes in body composition when weight is lost by diet alone versus diet plus exercise.
24. Describe the relationship of the fat-free mass and caloric intake to the BMR.
25. Define thermogenesis and how it is affected by both short-and long-term overfeeding.
26. Describe the effect of exercise on appetite and body composition.
27. Explain quantitatively why small differences in energy expenditure and dietary intake are important in weight gain over the years.

Multiple Choice

Instructions: After reading the question, and all possible answers, select the letter of choice that *BEST* answers the question. *Read all possible answers because some questions may have more than one correct answer.* The correct answers are provided at the end of this chapter.

1. Which of the following is *not* one of the U.S. Dietary Goals concerning caloric intake?
   a. increase carbohydrate intake to 55%-60%
   b. decrease fat consumption to 30%
   c. increase sugar consumption to 20%
   d. reduce salt consumption to 3 gm per day

2. Which of the following is a characteristic common to all vitamins?
   a. they are organic catalysts involved in metabolic reactions
   b. they are required in large amounts
   c. they are not degraded (metabolized) in the human body
   d. they are "used up" in metabolic reactions

3. Which of the following is *not* a fat soluble vitamin?
   a. Vitamin A
   b. Vitamin D
   c. Vitamin E
   d. Vitamin C

4. Which of the following is true of fat soluble vitamins?
   a. they can only be stored in small quantities in the body
   b. a deficiency state develops more quickly than for water-soluble vitamins
   c. so much can be stored in the body that a toxicity condition can occur
   d. None of the above.

5. Which of the following would be considered a major mineral?
   a. calcium
   b. iron
   c. zinc
   d. copper

6. Which of the following is a major function of calcium?
   a. component of enzymes
   b. body water balance
   c. nerve transmission
   d. Both a and c are correct.

7. Which of the following is a major function of sodium?
   a. body water balance
   b. nerve function
   c. blood clotting
   d. Both a and b are correct

8. Which of the following is a major function of iron?
   a. component of hemoglobin, myoglobin, and enzymes
   b. component of thyroid hormones
   c. maintenance of tooth structure
   d. formation of gastric juice

9. If an individual is diagnosed with anemia, they probably have a deficiency of
    a. calcium.
    b. iron.
    c. sodium.
    d. iodine.

10. Which of the following carbohydrates can be digested and metabolized for energy?
    a. sugars
    b. fiber
    c. cellulose
    d. hemicellulose

11. Starches are found in
    a. cereals.
    b. flour.
    c. potatoes.
    d. All of the above.

12. Which of the following depends exclusively on carbohydrate for its source of energy?
    a. red blood cells
    b. white blood cells
    c. liver cells
    d. skeletal muscle cells

13. A high fiber diet reduces the incidence of
    a. colon cancer.
    b. diverticulosis.
    c. stomach cancer.
    d. All of the above.

14. Which of the following is an *incorrect* statement about protein?
    a. provides 4 kcal per gram
    b. is a primary energy source
    c. is used for the synthesis of enzymes and hormones
    d. can be found in eggs, milk, and fish

15. Which food group has the highest recommended daily servings and can be found at the bottom of the food group pyramid?
    a. cereals
    b. fruit and vegetables
    c. meat and dairy products
    d. fats and oils

16. Which of the following procedures requires total body water to be determined in order to calculate body composition?
    a. skinfold thickness
    b. isotope dilution
    c. hydrostatic underwater weighing
    d. bioelectrical impedance analysis

17. When determining body composition via the technique of underwater weighing, Archimedes' principle is applied to determine the
    a. volume of the individual.
    b. density of the individual.
    c. weight of the individual.
    d. mass of the GI tract.

18. Which of the following diseases is obesity a primary contributing factor for?
    a. adult-onset diabetes
    b. endometrial carcinoma
    c. atherosclerotic disease
    d. gallbladder disease

19. Which of the following is true of low-carbohydrate, low calorie diets?
    a. they promote ketosis
    b. cause a rapid weight loss
    c. cause diuresis
    d. All of the above.

20. Basal Metabolic Rate is important in energy balance because it represents _____ of total energy expenditure in the average sedentary person.
    a. 60-75%
    b. 80%
    c. 75-90%
    d. 50-60%

21. Physical activity usually represents between _____ of daily energy expenditure
    a. 2-5%
    b. 5-10%
    c. 5-40%
    d. 50-60%

22. Women have a lower BMR due to
    a. higher fat-free mass.
    b. lower fat-free mass.
    c. thyroxine levels.
    d. None of the above.

23. The relationship between body fat and nonbasal energy expenditure is
    a. significant.
    b. non-significant.
    c. significant only in female.
    d. significant more in males.

24. For sedentary occupations, caloric intake exceeds needs and therefore
    a. body weight is increased.
    b. body weight is maintained.
    c. there is a loss in body weight.
    d. there is a loss in body weight then an increase.

25. When RQ>FQ
    a. the person is in nutrient balance.
    b. the person uses more fat than what is consumed.
    c. the person consumes more fat than what they use.
    d. None of the above.

True and False

Instructions: Read each question carefully and determine if the statement is true or false. The correct answers are provided at the end of this chapter.

1. The U.S. government established a set of dietary goals to improve health status.

2. Vitamin D is regarded as the most toxic of the fat-soluble vitamins.

3. Very few of the water-soluble vitamins are involved in energy metabolism.

4. Vitamin C is involved in the maintenance of bone, cartilage, and connective tissue.

5. Minerals are the chemical elements, other than carbon, hydrogen, oxygen, and nitrogen, associated with the structure and function of the body.

6. Deficient sodium intake can lead to hypertension in genetically susceptible individuals.

7. You would have to eat over three times as much fat as carbohydrate to consume the same number of calories.

8. Carbohydrate is a minor energy source for all tissues.

9. Dietary fiber cannot be digested and metabolized, and consequently provides a sense of fullness during a meal without the additional calories.

10. In the exchange system of planning a diet the caloric content and the percent of carbohydrate, fat, and protein in each food is the focus of attention.

11. When a person undergoes dietary restriction, the size of the fat cells decreases but the number does not.

12. A positive energy balance of 500 kcal per day would result in the gain of one pound per week.

13. Low-carbohydrate ketogenic diets can cause weakness, apathy, and fatigue.

14. The BMR is proportional to the fat-free mass, and after age 20 it decreases approximately 2% and 3% per decade in men and women respectively.

15. When RMR is expressed per unit of fat-free mass, there is a gender difference.

16. The heat generated due to the food we consume accounts for about 10%-15% of our total daily energy expenditure.

17. The advantage of using exercise compared to caloric restriction alone in weight-loss programs is that the composition of the weight that is lost is more fat tissue than lean tissue.

18. One of the major problems associated with height/weight tables is that there is no way to know the individuals body composition.

19. The most accurate way to measure body composition is via the skinfold technique.

20. Resting metabolic rate is not elevated following exercise.

21. Exercise is required to achieve weight loss.

22. Any form of exercise will contribute to fat loss.

23. Formerly sedentary individuals show a net increase in appetite when they undertake an exercise program.

24. Excess carbohydrate intake is converted to fat.

25. Alcohol suppresses fat oxidation.

Matching Terms and Definitions

Instructions: Consider each term carefully and select the correct definition below. There are two groups of terms and definitions for this chapter. The correct answers are provided at the end of the chapter.

Terms and Definitions (Group 1)

Terms (Group 1)
1. anorexia nervosa
2. basal metabolic rate (BMR)
3. bulimia nervosa
4. cholesterol
5. Daily Value (DV)
6. deficiency
7. Dietary Guidelines for Americans
8. elements
9. energy wasteful systems
10. ferritin
11. food records
12. HDL cholesterol
13. hemosiderin
14. high-density lipoproteins (HDL)
15. LDL cholesterol
16. lipoprotein

Definitions (Group 1)
a. A standard used in nutritional labeling.
b. A shortcoming of some essential nutrient.
c. A single chemical substance composed of only one type of atom.
d. Form of low-density lipoprotein responsible for the transport of plasma cholesterol.
e. An insoluble form of iron stored in tissues.
f. An eating disorder characterized by eating and forced regurgitation.
g. Proteins used to transport cholesterol in blood; high levels appear to offer some protection from atherosclerosis.
h. Metabolic pathways in which the energy generated in one reaction is used up in another, creating a futile cycle and requiring a higher resting metabolic rate.
i. A lipid that can be consumed in the diet or synthesized in cells and plays a role in the development of atherosclerosis.
j. Protein involved in the transport of cholesterol and triglycerides in the plasma.
k. Published in 1980 by the U.S. Departments of Agriculture.
l. Plasma protein that binds iron and is representative of the whole body iron store.
m. An eating disorder characterized by rapid weight loss due to failure to consume adequate amounts of nutrients.
n. The practice of keeping dietary food records for determining nutrient intake.
o. Cholesterol that is transported in the blood via high-density proteins; related to low risk of heart disease.
p. Metabolic rate measured in supine position following a twelve-hour fast, and eight hours of sleep.

Terms and Definitions (Group 2)

Terms (Group 2)

1. low-density lipoproteins (LDL)
2. major minerals
3. nutrient density
4. osteoporosis
5. provitamin
6. Recommended Dietary Allowances (RDA)
7. resting metabolic rate (RMR)
8. thermogenesis
9. toxicity
10. trace elements
11. transferrin
12. twenty-four-hour recall
13. underwater weighing
14. U.S. Dietary Goals
15. whole body density

Definitions (Group 2)

a. Calcium, phosphorus, potassium, sulfur, sodium, chloride, and magnesium.
b. A decrease in bone density due to a loss of cortical bone.
c. The generation of heat as a result of metabolic reactions.
d. Standards of nutrition associated with good health for the majority of people.
e. Form of lipoprotein that transports a majority of the plasma cholesterol.
f. The degree to which foods contain selected nutrients.
g. Procedure to estimate body volume by the loss of weight in water.
h. A precursor of a vitamin.
i. Metabolic rate measured in the supine position following a period of fasting (4-12 hours) and rest (4-8 hours).
j. A condition which can result from a chronic ingestion of vitamins.
k. Iron, zinc, copper, iodine, manganese, selenium, chromium, molybdenum, cobalt, arsenic, nickel, fluoride, and vanadium.
l. A technique of recording the type and amount of food consumed during a twenty-four-hour period.
m. A series of nutritional goals to achieve better health for the American population: 58% carbohydrate; 30% fat; and 12% protein.
n. A measure of the weight to volume ratio of the entire body; high values are associated with low body fatness.
o. The iron-carrying molecule used as an index of whole-body iron status.

Answers

Multiple Choice

1. c
2. a
3. d
4. c
5. a
6. c
7. d
8. a
9. b
10. a
11. d
12. a
13. b
14. b
15. a
16. b
17. a
18. a
19. d
20. a
21. c
22. b
23. a
24. a
25. c

True and False	Terms and Definitions (Group 1)	Terms and Definitions (Group 2)
1. True	1. m	1. e
2. True	2. p	2. a
3. False	3. f	3. f
4. True	4. i	4. b
5. True	5. a	5. h
6. False	6. b	6. d
7. False	7. k	7. i
8. False	8. c	8. c
9. True	9. h	9. j
10. True	10. l	10. k
11. True	11. n	11. o
12. True	12. o	12. l
13. True	13. e	13. g
14. True	14. g	14. m
15. False	15. d	15. n
16. True	16. j	
17. True		
18. True		
19. False		
20. False		
21. False		
22. True		
23. False		
24. False		
25. True		

Chapter 19: Factors Affecting Performance

Chapter Learning Objectives

After studying this chapter you should be able to do the following:

1. Identify factors affecting maximal performance.
2. Provide evidence for and against the central nervous system being a site of fatigue.
3. Identify potential neural factors in the periphery that may be linked to fatigue.
4. Explain the role of cross-bridge cycling in fatigue.
5. Summarize the evidence on the order of recruitment of muscle fibers with increasing intensities of activity, and the type of metabolism upon which each is dependent.
6. Describe the factors limiting performance in all-out activities lasting less than ten seconds.
7. Describe the factors limiting performance in all-out activities lasting 10-180 seconds.
8. Discuss the subtle changes in the factors affecting optimal performance as the duration of a maximal performance increases from three minutes to four hours.

Multiple Choice

Instructions: After reading the question, and all possible answers, select the letter of choice that *BEST* answers the question. *Read all possible answers because some questions may have more than one correct answer.* The correct answers are provided at the end of this chapter.

1. The central nervous system would be implicated in fatigue if there were _____ in the activity.
   a. an increase in number of functioning motor units
   b. a reduction in motor unit firing frequency
   c. an increase in motor unit firing frequency
   d. Both a and b are correct.

2. Fatigue due to neural factors could be associated with fatigue at the
   a. neuromuscular junction.
   b. sarcolemma.
   c. transverse tubules.
   d. All of the above.

3. One sign of fatigue in isometric contractions is a longer "relaxation time" which could be due to
   a. a faster cycling of the cross-bridge.
   b. pumping of Ca^{++} to the sarcoplasmic reticulum at a faster rate than normal.
   c. inadequate ATP.
   d. All of the above.

4. Which of the following is *not true* of Type IIa fibers?
   a. fatigue resistant
   b. recruited up to approximately 40% of VO_2 max
   c. fast-twitch
   d. dependent on oxygen delivery for tension development

5. Which of the following is true of Type IIb fibers?
   a. slow twitch
   b. can generate great tension via aerobic sources
   c. has a low mitochondrial content
   d. is recruited above approximately 40% VO_2 max

6. Ultra short-term performance (less than ten seconds) is limited by
   a. skill and technique.
   b. VO_2 max.
   c. mitochondrial and capillary density.
   d. maximal cardiac output.

7. Which of the following would *not* be a limiting factor in moderate-length performances (three to twenty minutes)?
   a. muscle fiber type
   b. dehydration
   c. VO_2 max
   d. maximal stroke volume

8. Which of the following would be a limiting factor to performance in a marathon?
   a. running economy
   b. steady state VO_2
   c. liver and muscle glycogen stores
   d. All of the above

9. Free radicals are
   a. highly reactive molecules.
   b. produced as a by-product of aerobic metabolism.
   c. can promote muscle fatigue.
   d. All of the above.

10. Which muscle fibers are recruited in the following order with increasing intensities of exercise?
    a. type I--> type IIa --> type IIb
    b. type IIb--> type IIa --> type I
    c. type IIa--> type I --> type IIb
    d. type I--> type IIb --> type IIa

True and False

Instructions: Read each question carefully and determine if the statement is true or false. The correct answers are provided at the end of the chapter.

1. Fatigue is defined as an inability to maintain a power output or force during repeated muscle contractions.

2. Scientists are in agreement about the exact cause of fatigue.

3. There is evidence both for and against the concept of "central fatigue".

4. Evidence shows that stimulating the muscle at a low frequency can lead to a slowing of the action potential waveform along the sarcolemma and the transverse tubules.

5. Exercise, especially eccentric exercise, can cause a physical disruption of the sarcomere, and increase the capacity of the muscle to produce tension.

6. A high H^+ concentration, due to a high rate of lactate formation, may interfere with Ca^{++} binding to troponin and reduce tension development.

7. Up to about 40% of VO_2 max, the Type I slow twitch oxidative muscle fiber is recruited to provide tension development.

8. Type I fibers have a great capacity to produce ATP via anaerobic glycolysis.

9. Maximal performances in the ten to sixty second range are still predominantly anaerobic.

10. As the duration of a performance increases, less demand is placed on the aerobic sources of energy.

11. Factors limiting performance in moderate-length races (three to twenty minutes) include the cardiovascular system and the mitochondrial content of the muscles involved in the activity.

12. The maximal stroke volume is crucial to a high cardiac output, and is influenced by both genetics and training.

13. During races between twenty and sixty minutes an individual who can run at a high percentage of VO_2 max would not have an advantage.

14. The longer the performance the greater the chance that environmental factors will play a role in the outcome.

15. Short-term explosive performances are dependent on Type IIb fibers and require a cardiovascular system that can deliver oxygen at a high rate to muscle fibers with many mitochondria.

Answers

Multiple Choice
1. b
2. d
3. c
4. b
5. c
6. a
7. b
8. d
9. a
10. d

True and False
1. True
2. False
3. True
4. False
5. False
6. True
7. True
8. False
9. True
10. False
11. True
12. True
13. False
14. True
15. False

Chapter 20: Work Tests to Evaluate Performance

Chapter Learning Objectives

After studying this chapter you should be able to do the following:

1. Discuss the rationale for the determination of VO_2 max in the evaluation of exercise performance in athletes competing in endurance events.
2. Explain the concept of "specificity of VO_2 max."
3. State the rationale for the assessment of the lactate threshold in the endurance athlete.
4. Discuss the purpose and technique(s) involved in the measurement of exercise economy.
5. Provide an overview of how laboratory tests performed on the endurance athlete might be interpreted as an aid in predicting performance.
6. Describe several tests that are useful in assessing anaerobic power.
7. Discuss the techniques used to evaluate strength.

Multiple Choice

Instructions: After reading the question, and all possible answers, select the letter of choice that *BEST* answers the question. *Read all possible answers because some questions may have more than one correct answer.* The correct answers are provided at the end of this chapter.

1. Why does an athlete undergo physiological testing in the laboratory?
   a. it identifies future Olympic gold medalists
   b. simulates the psychological demands of sports
   c. provides feedback of the effectiveness of a training program
   d. simulates the physiological demands of sports

2. In order for laboratory testing to be effective, several key factors need consideration. Which of the following is true?
   a. tests should be repeated regularly
   b. tests should be valid and reliable
   c. tests should be as sport specific as possible
   d. All of the above.

3. What are the two most common forms of exercise used to determine VO_2 max?
   a. running on treadmill and pedaling on a cycle ergometer
   b. walking on treadmill and pedaling on a cycle ergometer
   c. pedaling on a cycle ergometer and arm ergometry
   d. swimming and walking on treadmill

4. What is the primary criterion used to determine if VO_2 max has been reached during an incremental exercise test?
   a. a plateau in oxygen uptake with a further increase in work rate
   b. a respiratory exchange ratio > 1.15
   c. $\pm$ 10 beats/min. within predicted max heart rate
   d. None of the above.

5. Which of the following is the most common laboratory measurement to estimate maximal steady state speed?
   a. VO_2 max
   b. ventilatory threshold
   c. lactate threshold
   d. None of the above.

6. When oxygen uptake is graphed as a function of running speed, runner B requires less oxygen than runner A at any given running speed. Based on this information which of the following is true?
   a. runner B expends more energy than runner A
   b. runner A is more economical than runner B
   c. runner B is more economical than runner A
   d. runner A has a lower lactate threshold than runner B

7. Which of the following is *not* a test of ultra short-term maximal anaerobic power?
   a. Wingate test
   b. Margaria power test
   c. Sargent's jump and reach test
   d. standing long jump

8. Which of the following tests was developed in 1983 to assess ultra short-term anaerobic power in cyclists?
   a. Margaria power test
   b. Wingate test
   c. isometric assessment of strength
   d. Quebec 10-second test

9. Which of the following must be considered when selecting a method to test strength for a specific sport?
   a. movement pattern
   b. contraction type
   c. velocity of the contraction
   d. All of the above.

10. Which of the following is an advantage of isometric testing using computerized equipment?
    a. safe to administer
    b. inexpensive
    c. allows dynamic movements
    d. minimal time required to perform the test

11. Which of the following is a disadvantage of isotonic strength testing?
    a. high cost of equipment
    b. force is not dynamically applied
    c. possibility of subject injury using 1-RM
    d. All of the above.

12. The cable tensiometer is a tension-measuring device, and was one of the first techniques used to measure
    a. isometric strength.
    b. isotonic strength.
    c. dynamic strength.
    d. None of the above.

13. A laboratory measure that can be used to predict performance in endurance events is
    a. Sargent's jump and reach test.
    b. Margaria power test.
    c. Wingate test.
    d. critical power test.

14. The relationship between running peak velocity and finish time for a 5 kilometer race is
    a. exponential.
    b. linear.
    c. j shape.
    d. curvilinear.

15. Ultra short tern tests attempts to determine the maximal capacity of the
    a. ATP-PC system.
    b. anaerobic glycolysis system.
    c. aerobic system.
    d. Both a and b are correct.

True and False

Instructions: Read each question carefully and determine if the statement is true or false. The correct answers are provided at the end of the chapter.

1. A test that stresses the same physiological systems required by a particular sport or athletic event would appear to be a valid means of assessing physical performance.

2. Relative VO_2 max has been shown to be the single most important factor in predicting distance running success in a heterogeneous (i.e., different VO_2 max) group of athletes.

3. The correlation between VO_2 max and distance running performance is low in a homogeneous (i.e., similar VO_2 max) group of runners.

4. When testing untrained subjects, a plateau in VO_2 is often observed during an incremental exercise test.

5. The highest VO_2 obtained during an incremental arm ergometry test is referred to as VO_2 max.

6. A runner who is uneconomical will expend a greater amount of energy to run at a given speed than an economical runner.

7. Numerous studies have shown that a close relationship exists between the lactate or ventilatory threshold and the maximal pace that can be maintained during a 10,000-meter race.

8. The Margaria power test has been shown to be a poor predictor of success in a 40-yard dash.

9. The Sargent's jump-and-reach test and the standing long jump probably fail to adequately assess an individual's maximal ATP-PC system capacity because of the brief duration of each test.

10. The technical error of the Quebec 10-second test is small and the procedure is highly reliable.

11. The Wingate test offers an excellent means of evaluating anaerobic power output in cyclists.

12. Muscular strength is the maximum force that can be generated by a muscle or muscle group.

13. Muscular strength can be evaluated using a variable resistance machine.

14. The advantages of isokinetic strength testing is the low cost of equipment.

15. The incidence of injury increases when using a 3-RM test compared to a 1-RM test.

Matching Terms and Definitions

Instructions: Consider each term carefully and select the correct definition below. The correct answers are provided at the end of the chapter.

Terms
1. critical power
2. dynamometer
3. isokinetic
4. Margaria power test
5. muscular strength
6. power tests
7. Quebec 10-second test
8. Sargent's jump-and-reach test
9. Wingate test

Definitions
a. The running speed at which the running speed/time curve reaches a plateau.
b. A test measuring the quantity of work accomplished in a time period.
c. A test of anaerobic power dependent on the high-energy phosphates; a vertical jump test.
d. Test of anaerobic power, primarily related to high-energy phosphates, in which a subject runs up stairs with time monitored to the nearest hundredth of a second.
e. Anaerobic power test to evaluate maximal rate at which glycolysis can deliver ATP.
f. Action in which the rate of movement is constantly maintained through a specific range of motion even though maximal force is exerted.
g. The maximal amount of force that can be generated by a muscle or muscle group.
h. Device used to measure force production.
i. A maximal effort 10-second cycle test designed to assess ultra short-term anaerobic power during cycling.

Answers

Multiple Choice	True and False	Terms and Definitions
1. a	1. True	1. a
1. c	2. True	2. h
2. d	3. True	3. f
3. a	4. False	4. d
4. a	5. False	5. g
5. c	6. True	6. b
6. c	7. True	7. i
7. a	8. False	8. c
8. d	9. True	9. e
9. d	10. True	
10. a	11. True	
11. c	12. True	
12. a	13. True	
13. d	14. False	
14. b	15. False	
15. a		

Chapter 21: Training for Performance

Chapter Learning Objectives

After studying this chapter you should be able to do the following:

1. Discuss the concept of designing a sport-specific training program based on an analysis of the energy systems utilized by the activity.
2. List and discuss the general principles of physical conditioning for improved sport performance.
3. Define the terms *overload, specificity,* and *reversibility.*
4. Outline the use of interval training and continuous training in the improvement of the maximal aerobic power in athletes.
5. Discuss the guidelines associated with planning a training program designed to improve the anaerobic power of athletes.
6. Outline the principles of training for the improvement of strength.
7. Discuss the role of gender differences in the development of strength.
8. List the factors that contribute to delayed onset muscle soreness.
9. Discuss the use of static and ballistic stretching to improve flexibility.
10. Outline the goals of: 1) off-season conditioning, 2) preseason conditioning, and 3) in-season conditioning.
11. List and discuss several common training errors.

Multiple Choice

Instructions: After reading the question, and all possible answers, select the letter of choice that *BEST* answers the question. *Read all possible answers because some questions may have more than one correct answer.* The correct answers are provided at the end of this chapter.

1. Training programs need to deal with specificity by using the
   a. muscle groups that will be used in competition.
   b. energy systems that will provide the energy in competition.
   c. muscle groups and energy systems not used during competition.
   d. Both a and b are correct.

2. Many factors contribute to the observed individual variations in the training response. Which of the following would be considered the most important?
   a. genetics
   b. athlete's beginning level of fitness
   c. gender
   d. race

3. Which of the following would *not* occur during warm-up exercises?
   a. decreased enzyme activity in skeletal muscle
   b. increased blood flow to skeletal muscle
   c. increase in muscle temperature
   d. increased cardiac output

4. What is the principle objective of the "cool down"?
   a. improve flexibility
   b. return blood pressure to normal
   c. return "pooled" blood from the exercised muscle back to central circulation
   d. return heart rate to normal

5. In training to improve aerobic power, the work interval should generally last longer than
   a. 30 seconds.
   b. 40 seconds.
   c. 50 seconds.
   d. 60 seconds.

6. Recent evidence suggests that _____ is superior to long term low intensity exercise in improving VO_2 max.
   a. short-term high-intensity exercise
   b. long-term high intensity exercise
   c. short-term low intensity exercise
   d. Any of the above.

7. The exact intensity that elicits greatest improvement in VO_2 max is
   a. unknown at present.
   b. 70% of VO_2 max.
   c. 80% of VO_2 max.
   d. 90% of VO_2 max.

8. A recent review of exercise-training-induced injuries suggests that the majority of training injuries are a result of
   a. footwear problems.
   b. overtraining.
   c. musculotendonous imbalance of strength and/or flexibility.
   d. poor running surface.

9. After approximately ten seconds of a maximal effort, there is a growing dependence on energy production from
   a. ATP-PC system.
   b. electron transport chain.
   c. anaerobic glycolysis.
   d. oxidative phosphorylation.

10. Which energy system provides most of the energy for the 40-yard dash?
    a. ATP-PC system
    b. anaerobic glycolysis
    c. oxidative phosphorylation
    d. None of the above.

11. Which of the following is not part of the proposed model for the occurrence of delayed onset muscle soreness?
    a. structural damage to muscle cells
    b. protease activation results in synthesis of cellular proteins
    c. calcium leakage out of sarcoplasmic reticulum
    d. inflammatory response

12. Of the following athletes, which would need to be the least flexible for optimum performance in their sport?
    a. gymnast
    b. tennis player
    c. football player
    d. ballet dancer

13. Which of the following training regimes is composed of low-intensity, high-volume work?
    a. off-season training
    b. preseason training
    c. inseason training
    d. All of the above.

14. Which of the following is not a general symptom of overtraining?
    a. chronic fatigue
    b. psychological staleness
    c. multiple sore throats
    d. weight gain

15. Which of the following is not a common mistake of training?
    a. undertraining
    b. overtraining
    c. tapering
    d. non-specific exercises

True and False

Instructions: Read each question carefully and determine if the statement is true or false. The correct answers are provided at the end of the chapter.

1. Men and women respond to training programs in a dissimilar fashion.

2. Training to improve endurance performance should be geared toward increasing the lactate threshold, and improving VO_2 max and running economy.

3. In general, exercise heart rates should reach 85%-100% of the maximal heart rate during interval training.

4. Blood pressure appears to be the most practical means of evaluating exercise intensity during training.

5. Isometric exercise is the application of force without joint movement.

6. Staron and colleagues demonstrated that twenty weeks of high-intensity strength training resulted in a conversion of type IIa to type IIb fibers in college age females.

7. Strength gains increase when the number of repetitions are greater than fifteen.

8. The speed of muscle shortening during training should be similar to those speeds used during the event.

9. Athletes who perform strength and endurance training programs on the same day show less strength gain compared to athletes performing strength training alone.

10. The sex difference in strength is eliminated when force production in men and women is compared on the basis of the cross-sectional area of muscle.

Matching Terms and Definitions

Instructions: Consider each term carefully and select the correct definition below. The correct answers are provided at the end of the chapter.

Terms
1. delayed onset muscle soreness (DOMS)
2. dynamic stretching
3. hyperplasia
4. hypertrophy
5. progressive resistance exercise (PRE)
6. proprioceptive neuromuscular facilitation
7. repetition
8. rest interval
9. set
10. static stretching
11. tapering
12. variable resistance exercise
13. work interval

Definitions
a. A basic unit of a workout containing the number of times a specific exercise is done.
b. The number of times an exercise is repeated within a single exercise "set".
c. Stretching procedure in which a muscle is stretched and held in the stretched position for ten to thirty seconds.
d. Stretching that involves controlled movement.
e. An increase in the number of cells in a tissue.
f. In interval training, the duration of the work phase of each work-to-rest interval.
g. A training program in which the muscles must work against a gradually increasing resistance.
h. Technique of preceding a static stretch with an isometric contraction.
i. Muscle soreness that occurs twelve to twenty-four hours after an exercise bout.
j. The time period between bouts in an interval training program.
k. Strength training equipment in which the resistance varies throughout the range of motion.
l. An increase in cell size.
m. Reducing training load several days before a performance.

Answers

Multiple Choice	True and False	Terms and Definitions
1. d	1. F	1. i
2. b	2. T	2. d
3. a	3. T	3. e
4. c	4. F	4. l
5. d	5. T	5. g
6. a	6. F	6. h
7. a	7. F	7. b
8. b	8. T	8. j
9. c	9. T	9. a
10. a	10. T	10. c
11. b		11. m
12. c		12. k
13. a		13. f
14. d		
15. c		

Chapter 22: Training for Special Populations

Chapter Learning Objectives

After studying this chapter you should be able to do the following:

1. Describe the incidence of amenorrhea in female athletes versus the general population.
2. List those factors thought to contribute to "athletic" amenorrhea.
3. Discuss the general recommendations for training during menstruation.
4. List the general guidelines for exercise during pregnancy.
5. Define the term "female athlete triad."
6. Discuss the possibility that chronic exercise presents a danger to: 1) the cardiopulmonary system, or 2) the musculoskeletal system of children.
7. List those conditions in Type I diabetes that might limit their participation in a vigorous training program.
8. Explain the rationale for the selection of an insulin injection site for Type I diabetes prior to a training session.
9. List the precautions that should be taken by asthmatics during a training session.
10. Discuss the question "Does exercise promote seizures in epileptics?"

Multiple Choice

Instructions: After reading the question, and all possible answers, select the letter of choice that *BEST* answers the question. *Read all possible answers because some questions may have more than one correct answer.* The correct answers are provided at the end of this chapter.

1. Insulin injected subcutaneously in the leg prior to running (or other forms of leg exercise) could result in
   a. exercise-induced hyperglycemia.
   b. exercise-induced hypoglycemia.
   c. decreased glucose uptake by the muscle.
   d. increased glucose release from the liver.

2. Current knowledge concerning training for children is limited primarily to
   a. mitochondria and oxidative enzymes.
   b. skeletal muscle.
   c. the cardiopulmonary system.
   d. None of the above.

3. Where is growth cartilage found?
   a. epiphyseal plate
   b. articular cartilage
   c. apophyses
   d. All of the above.

4. Which of the following activities can cause can cause premature closure of the growth plate and retard normal long bone growth in children?
   a. swimming
   b. basketball
   c. strength training
   d. track and field

5. The occurrence of amenorrhea is rather high in
   a. swimming.
   b. cycling.
   c. ballet dancing.
   d. None of the above.

6. Why has it been recommended that pregnant women engage in swimming?
   a. accelerated heat transfer
   b. support for body weight
   c. the most dramatic fitness gains are achieved with swimming
   d. Both a and b are correct.

7. What causes menstrual cycle dysfunction in athletes ?
   a. low body fat
   b. hormonal alterations
   c. psychological stress
   d. All of the above.

8. The release of prostaglandins begins
   a. just prior to the onset of menstrual flow.
   b. just after the onset of menstrual flow.
   c. during menstrual flow.
   d. two to three days after the onset of menstrual flow.

9. Major cause/s of bone loss in female athletes is/are
   a. estrogen deficiency due to amenorrhea.
   b. inadequate calcium intake.
   c. low body fat.
   d. Both a and b are correct.

10. Which of the following should be avoided during pregnancy?
    a. short term-low intensity exercise
    b. light resistance training
    c. high intensity training
    d. All of the above.

True and False

Instructions: Read each question carefully and determine if the statement is true or false. The correct answers to this exam are provided at the end of the chapter.

1. Type II diabetics are more likely to engage in training for performance purposes than Type I diabetes.

2. The key to safe participation in sport conditioning for the diabetic athlete is to learn to avoid hypoglycemic episodes during training.

3. The site of insulin injection should be close to the working muscle.

4. Young diabetics respond to a conditioning program in a manner similar to healthy children.

5. Division exists in the medical community concerning the risk of exercise and epileptic seizures.

6. Children appear to adapt to endurance training at a much faster rate than adults.

7. Amenorrhea in athletes appears to be related to training intensity.

8. The incidence of amenorrhea in the general population is approximately 3%, while the incidence in distance runners is 24%.

Matching Terms and Definitions

Instructions: Consider each term carefully and select the correct definition below. The correct answers are provided at the end of the chapter.

Terms
1. amenorrhea
2. apophyses
3. articular cartilage
4. dysmenorrhea
5. epilepsy
6. epiphyseal plate (growth plate)

Definitions
a. A neurological disorder manifested by muscular seizures.
b. Cartilage that covers the end of bones in a synovial joint.
c. The absence of menses.
d. Cartilaginous layer between the head and shaft of a long bone where growth takes place.
e. Sites of muscle-tendon insertion in bones.
f. Painful menstruation.

Answers

Multiple Choice	True and False	Terms and Definitions
1. b	1. F	1. c
2. c	2. T	2. e
3. d	3. F	3. b
4. c	4. T	4. f
5. c	5. T	5. a
6. d	6. F	6. d
7. d	7. T	
8. a	8. T	
9. d		
10. c		

Chapter 23: Nutrition, Body Composition, and Performance

Chapter Learning Objectives

After studying this chapter you should be able to do the following:

1. Describe the effect of various carbohydrate diets on muscle glycogen and on endurance performance during heavy exercise.
2. Contrast the "classic" method of achieving a supercompensation of the muscle glycogen stores with the "modified" method.
3. Describe some potential problems when glucose is ingested immediately prior to exercise.
4. Describe the importance of blood glucose as a fuel in prolonged exercise, and the role of carbohydrate supplementation during the performance.
5. Contrast the evidence that protein is oxidized at a faster rate during exercise with the evidence that the use of labeled amino acids may be an inappropriate methodology to study this issue.
6. Describe the need for protein *during* the adaptation to a new, more strenuous exercise level with the protein need when the adaptation is complete.
7. Defend the recommendation that a protein intake that is 12%-15% of energy intake is sufficient to meet an athlete's demand.
8. Describe the recommended fluid replacement strategies for athletic events of different intensities and durations, citing evidence to support your position.
9. Describe the salt requirement of the athlete, compared to the sedentary individual, and the recommended means of maintaining sodium balance.
10. List the steps leading to iron deficiency anemia and the special problem that athletes have in maintaining iron balance.
11. Provide a brief summary of the effects of vitamin supplementation on performance.
12. Characterize the role of the pregame meal on performance and the rationale for limiting fats and proteins.
13. Describe the various components of the somatotype and what the following ratings signify: 171, 711, and 117.
14. Describe what the endomorphic and mesomorphic components in the Heath-Carter method of somatotyping represent in conventional body composition analysis.
15. Explain why one must be careful in recommending specific body fatness values for individual athletes.

Multiple Choice

Instructions: After reading the question, and all possible answers, select the letter of choice that *BEST* answers the question. *Read all possible answers because some questions may have more than one correct answer.* The correct answers are provided at the end of this chapter.

1. Muscle glycogen has been shown to be systematically depleted during
   a. slow walking.
   b. heavy exercise (77% VO_2 max).
   c. the 100 meter sprint.
   d. field events e.g. high jump.

2. It has been shown that time to exhaustion during heavy exercise can be delayed by
   a. consuming large amounts of glucose just prior to exercise.
   b. manipulating the quantity of fat in the diet.
   c. manipulating the quantity of carbohydrate in the diet.
   d. All of the above are true.

3. The limiting factor in muscle glycogen synthesis is
   a. glucose transport across the cell membrane.
   b. the activity of glycogen synthase.
   c. the activity of phosphofructokinase.
   d. the activity of phosphorylase.

4. Which of the following is/are superior for synthesizing muscle glycogen
   a. glucose.
   b. fructose.
   c. glucose polymers.
   d. Both a and c are superior.

5. The ingestion of carbohydrate during prolonged moderate exercise appears to
   a. spare muscle glycogen.
   b. spare liver glycogen.
   c. stimulate gluconeogenesis.
   d. Both a and b are correct.

6. Which of the following statements concerning glucose polymer solutions is false?
   a. they help to maintain blood glucose concentration during exercise
   b. palatability is improved if carbohydrate concentrations are above 10%
   c. if blood glucose is maintained the exercising subject will not fatigue
   d. they are used frequently in events such as the marathon

7. The adult RDA for protein is easily met by a diet having _____ of its energy as protein.
   a. 5%
   b. 12%
   c. 2%
   d. 8%

8. When an individual excretes less nitrogen than he/she consumes it is called
   a. nitrogen balance.
   b. nitrogen excretion.
   c. positive nitrogen balance.
   d. negative nitrogen balance.

9. Which of the following statements concerning oxidation of amino acids is false?
   a. muscle releases alanine in proportion to exercise intensity
   b. nitrogen derived from leucine can be found in plasma urea
   c. alanine is used in the liver for gluconeogenesis
   d. catabolism of protein is higher during exercise than rest

10. The primary mechanism for heat loss at high work rates in a comfortable environment is
    a. conduction.
    b. convection.
    c. radiation.
    d. evaporation of sweat.

11. Which of the following has been shown to delay gastric emptying?
    a. low body temperature
    b. dehydration
    c. euhydration
    d. hyperhydration

12. During exercise lasting less than one hour (80%-130% VO$_2$ max) the athlete should drink
    a. 500-1,000 ml of water.
    b. 10-20 mEq of Na$^+$ and Cl$^-$ and 6%-8% carbohydrate.
    c. 12% glucose-polymer drink.
    d. 200 ml of water.

13. Which of the following is the most common nutritional deficiency?
    a. iron deficiency
    b. vitamin C deficiency
    c. calcium deficiency
    d. protein deficiency

14. Which of the following statements concerning a "recovery drink" is false?
    a. the addition of salt promotes fluid absorption
    b. the addition of salt promotes carbohydrate absorption
    c. the addition of salt replenishes some of the electrolytes
    d. the addition of salt reduces the palatability

15. The primary nutrient in the pregame meal should be
    a. simple carbohydrates.
    b. complex carbohydrates.
    c. fat.
    d. protein.

16. The pregame meal should be eaten
    a. about three hours prior to competition.
    b. 30 min. prior to competition .
    c. one hour prior to competition.
    d. five hours prior to competition.

17. According to Sheldon, an individual classified as a mesomorph would display
    a. a relative predominance of soft roundness.
    b. a relative predominance of muscle, bone and connective tissue.
    c. a relative predominance of linearity and fragility.
    d. a large surface area to mass ratio.

18. Somatotype considers
    a. body form.
    b. body shape.
    c. body size.
    d. Both a and b are correct.

19. A 171 somatotype rating would signify
    a. a primary endomorph.
    b. a primary mesomorph.
    c. a primary ectomorph.
    d. None of the above.

20. During exercise lasting less than one hour an athlete should drink
    a. 5-10 ml of water.
    b. 50-100 ml of water.
    c. 500-1000 ml of water.
    d. 5-10 liters of water.

True and False

Instructions: Read each question carefully and determine if the statement is true or false. The correct answers to this exam are provided at the end of the chapter.

1. Time to exhaustion is directly related to the initial glycogen store in the working muscles.

2. It takes about ten hours to replenish muscle glycogen following prolonged moderate exercise, provided that about 200-300 gms of carbohydrate are ingested.

3. Following a bout of heavy exercise there is a decrease in the muscles sensitivity to insulin.

4. Hypoglycemia results when the rate of blood glucose uptake is not matched by release from the liver and/or small intestine.

5. The pre-exercise feeding should contain between one and five gm of carbohydrate per kilogram of body weight.

6. The ingestion of carbohydrate appears to spare the liver glycogen store by directly contributing carbohydrate for oxidation.

7. If a person becomes sodium depleted, body water increases, and the risk of heat injury increases.

8. A trained individual loses more Na^+ in sweat than an untrained person.

9. Inadequate intake of dietary iron has been cited as a primary cause of iron deficiency in women athletes.

10. A distance runner would be more ectomorphic than a weight lifter.

11. In a sport or activity where body weight must be carried along, (running or jumping) there is a positive correlation between body fatness and performance.

Matching Terms and Definitions

Instructions: Consider each term carefully and select the correct definition below. The corrects answers are provided at the end of the chapter.

Terms
1. ectomorphy
2. endomorphy
3. glucose polymer
4. mesomorphy
5. somatotype
6. supercompensation

Definitions
a. One component of a somatotype that characterizes the muscular form or lean body mass aspect of the human body.
b. A complex sugar molecule that contains multiple simple sugar molecules linked together.
c. An increase in the muscle glycogen content above normal levels following an exercise-induced muscle glycogen depletion and an increase in carbohydrate intake.

d. Body-type classification method used to characterize the degree to which an individual's frame is linear, muscular, and round.
e. The somatotype category that is rated for roundness (fatness).
f. Category of somatotype that is rated for linearity of body form.

Answers

Multiple Choice	True and False	Terms and Definitions
1. b	1. True	1. f
2. c	2. False	2. e
3. a	3. False	3. b
4. d	4. True	4. a
5. b	5. True	5. d
6. c	6. True	6. c
7. b	7. False	
8. c	8. False	
9. b	9. True	
10. d	10. True	
11. b	11. False	
12. a		
13. a		
14. d		
15. b		
16. a		
17. b		
18. d		
17. b		
18. d		
19. b		
20. c		

Chapter 24: Exercise and the Environment

Chapter Learning Objectives

After studying this chapter you should be able to do the following:

1. Describe the changes in atmospheric pressure (PO_2), air temperature, and air density with increasing altitude.
2. Describe how altitude affects sprint performances and explain why that is the case.
3. Explain why distance running performance decreases at high altitude.
4. Draw a graph to show the effect of altitude on VO_2 max and list the reasons for this response.
5. Graphically describe the effect of altitude on the heart rate and ventilation responses to submaximal work, and offer an explanation of why these changes are appropriate.
6. Describe the process of adaptation to altitude, and the degree to which this adaptation can be complete.
7. Explain why such variability exists among athletes in the decrease in VO_2 max upon exposure to altitude, the degree of improvement in VO_2 max at altitude, and the gains made upon return to sea level.
8. Describe the potential problems associated with training at high altitude and how one might get around them.
9. Explain the circumstances that caused physiologists to reevaluate their conclusions that humans could not climb Mount Everest without oxygen.
10. Explain the role that hyperventilation plays in helping to maintain a high oxygen-hemoglobin saturation at extreme altitudes.
11. List and describe the factors influencing the risk of heat injury.
12. Provide suggestions for the fitness participant to follow to minimize the likelihood of heat injury.
13. Describe in general terms the guidelines suggested for running road races in the heat.
14. Describe the three elements in the heat stress index, and explain why one is more important than the other two.
15. List the factors influencing hypothermia.
16. Explain what the Wind-chill Index is relative to convective heat loss.
17. Explain why exposure to cold water is more dangerous than exposure of air to the same temperature.
18. Describe what the clo unit is and how recommendations for insulation change when one does exercise.
19. Describe the role of subcutaneous fat and energy production in the development of hypothermia.
20. List the steps to follow to deal with hypothermia.
21. Explain how carbon monoxide can influence performance, and list the steps that should be taken to reduce the impact of pollution on performance.

Multiple Choice

Instructions: After reading the question, and all possible answers, select the letter of choice that *BEST* answers the question. *Read all possible answers because some questions may have more than one correct answer.* The correct answers are provided at the end of this chapter.

1. Which of the following statements is false?
   a. atmospheric pressure decreases with increasing altitude
   b. the air is less dense at high altitudes compared to sea level
   c. the percentage of oxygen in the air decreases with increasing altitude
   d. each liter of air contains fewer molecules of gas at increasing altitude

2. Which of the following events would be most likely to suffer when competing at high altitude?
   a. long jump
   b. high jump
   c. 400 meters
   d. marathon

3. With increasing altitude VO_2 max
   a. decreases in a linear fashion.
   b. decreases in a non linear fashion.
   c. increases in a linear fashion.
   d. does not change.

4. If VO_2 max decreases with increasing altitude, and maximal stroke volume and maximal heart rate do not change, then the decrease in VO_2 max must be due to
   a. decreased maximal cardiac output.
   b. decreased oxygen extraction at the muscle.
   c. an increased arteriovenous oxygen difference.
   d. All of the above.

5. What will happen to submaximal heart rate during exercise at altitude for any given level of submaximal oxygen consumption when compared to sea level?
   a. increase
   b. decrease
   c. remain the same
   d. depends on the type of activity

6. In order to have complete adaptation to high altitude one must
   a. spend the developmental years at high altitude.
   b. have been born at high altitude.
   c. spend at least 3 months at high altitude.
   d. spend at least 4 years at high altitude.

7. Which of the following is a physiological change that has been shown to occur as a result of exposure to extreme altitudes?
   a. increases in muscle fiber area
   b. increases in mitochondrial volume
   c. decreases in muscle fiber area
   d. Both a and b are correct.

8. The arterial saturation of hemoglobin is dependent upon
   a. arterial PO_2.
   b. arterial PCO_2.
   c. arterial pH.
   d. All of the above.

9. A low PCO_2 and a high pH
   a. causes the oxygen hemoglobin curve to shift to the left.
   b. causes the oxygen hemoglobin curve to shift to the right.
   c. results in increased saturation of hemoglobin.
   d. Both a and c are correct.

10. It has been shown that those who successfully deal with altitude have
    a. weak hypoxic ventilatory drives.
    b. lower arterial PO_2.
    c. strong hypoxic ventilatory drives.
    d. the ability to hypoventilate.

11. Which of the following statements is false?
    a. frequent exercise in the heat increases the capacity to sweat and reduces salt loss
    b. inadequate hydration reduces sweat rate and increases the chance of heat injury
    c. evaporation of sweat is dependent on a temperature gradient from skin to environment
    d. wind will increase the rate of heat loss by convection

12. The heart rate is a sensitive indicator of
    a. dehydration.
    b. environmental heat load.
    c. acclimatization.
    d. All of the above.

13. Which of the following is not one of the recommendations in the ACSM position stand on The Prevention of Thermal Injuries During Distance Running?
    a. plan races for the cooler months
    b. have a water station every 8-10 km
    c. encourage runner to drink 100-200 milliliters of water per water station
    d. provide medical facilities at race site to provide first aid

14. In order to quantify the overall heat stress associated with any environment, a _____ guide was developed.
    a. Wet Bulb Globe Temperature
    b. Dry Bulb Temperature
    c. Black Globe Temperature
    d. White Globe Temperature

15. What is the term for a higher rate of heat loss from the body compared to heat production?
    a. hypoxia
    b. hypothermia
    c. hyperthermia
    d. thermia

16. When the temperature is -4 degrees Celsius
    a. a minimal amount of heat is lost through the head.
    b. most of the heat loss occurs via the torso.
    c. about half of the heat is lost through the head.
    d. most of the heat loss occurs through the extremities.

17. Which of the following is not a recommended treatment for a person suffering from hypothermia?
    a. leave wet clothing on
    b. provide warm drinks
    c. keep the person awake
    d. put them into a sleeping bag

18. Which of the following pollutants does not affect lung function in normal adults, but causes bronchoconstriction in asthmatics?
    a. ozone
    b. sulfur dioxide
    c. carbon monoxide
    d. None of the above.

19. Carbon monoxide affects performance by
    a. depressing respiratory function.
    b. reducing oxygen transport.
    c. increasing carbon dioxide concentration.
    d. none of the above.

20. Increasing ozone concentration affects performance by
    a. depressing respiratory function.
    b. reducing oxygen transport.
    c. increasing carbon dioxide concentration.
    d. None of the above.

True and False

Instructions: Read each question carefully and determine if the statement is true or false. The correct answers to this exam are provided at the end of the chapter.

1. In addition to the hypoxic condition at altitude, the air temperature and humidity are lower.

2. The density of the air at altitude offers more resistance to movements at high speeds.

3. The capacity to transport oxygen to the working muscles at high altitude is reduced due to desaturation.

4. A variety of studies have shown a decrease in maximal heart rate at high altitude.

5. The average person who participates in an exercise program will have to increase the intensity of exercise at altitude in order to stay in the target heart rate zone.

6. Pulmonary ventilation increases with increasing altitudes.

7. VO_2 max decreases with increasing altitude due to the lower barometric pressure, which causes a lower PO_2 and a desaturation of hemoglobin.

8. The environmental temperature needs to be below freezing to cause hypothermia.

9. The rate of heat loss at any given temperature is indirectly influenced by the wind speed.

10. Wind is the only factor that can increase the rate of heat loss at any given temperature.

11. The thermal conductivity of water is about twenty-five times greater than that of air so you can lose heat faster in water than in air.

12. At low environmental temperatures the water vapor pressure is low even when the relative humidity is high.

Matching Terms and Definitions

Instructions: Consider each term carefully and select the correct definition. The correct answers are provided at the end of the chapter.

Terms
1. clo
2. hypoxia
3. hyperoxia
4. normoxia

Definitions
a. A relative lack of oxygen.
b. A normal PO_2.
c. Unit that describes the insulation quality of clothing.
d. Oxygen concentration in an inspired gas that exceeds 21%.

Answers

Multiple Choice
1. c
2. d
3. a
4. b
5. a
6. a
7. c
8. d
9. d
10. c
11. c
12. d
13. b
14. a
15. b
16. c
17. d
18. b
17. d
18. b
19. b
20. a

True and False
1. True
2. False
3. True
4. True
5. False
6. True
7. True
8. False
9. False
10. False
11. True
12. True

Terms and Definitions
1. c
2. a
3. d
4. b

Chapter 25: Ergogenic Aids

Chapter Learning Objectives

After studying this chapter you should be able to do the following:

1. Define ergogenic aid.
2. Explain why a "placebo" treatment in a "double-blind design" is used in research studies involving ergogenic aids.
3. Describe, in general, the effectiveness of nutritional supplements on performance.
4. Describe the effect of additional oxygen on performance; distinguish between hyperbaric oxygenation and that accomplished by breathing oxygen-enriched gas mixtures.
5. Describe the effect of additional oxygen performance: distinguish between hyperbaric oxygenation and that accomplished by breathing oxygen-enriched gas mixtures.
6. Describe blood doping and its potential for improving endurance performance.
7. Explain the mechanism by which ingested buffers might improve anaerobic performances.
8. Explain how amphetamines might improve exercise performance.
9. Describe the various mechanisms by which caffeine might improve performance.
10. Identify the risks associated with using chewing tobacco to obtain a nicotine "high".
11. Describe the risks of cocaine use and how it can cause death.
12. Describe the physiological and psychological effects of different types of warm-up.

Multiple Choice

Instructions: After reading the question, and all possible answers, select the letter of choice that *BEST* answers the question. *Read all possible answers because some questions may have more than one correct answer.* The correct answers are provided at the end of this chapter.

1. A placebo is a/an
   a. substance that will influence performance.
   b. a "look -alike" substance that will not influence performance.
   c. ergogenic aid.
   d. None of the above.

2. Which of the following terms best describes a research design in which neither the subject nor the investigator knows who is receiving the placebo or the substance under investigation?
   a. triple-blind research design
   b. blind research design
   c. double-blind research design
   d. independent scientific investigation

3. Which of the following statements is true?
   a. oxygen breathing before performance improves endurance performance
   b. oxygen breathing after performance improves endurance performance
   c. oxygen breathing during exercise improves endurance performance
   d. All of the above are true.

4. Elevations in the $[H^+]$ in muscle can decrease the activity of phosphofructokinase (PFK) which may
   a. activate glycolysis.
   b. increase Ca^{++} efflux from the terminal cisternae.
   c. increase the binding of calcium to troponin.
   d. interfere with excitation-contraction coupling.

5. The primary means by which H$^+$ is buffered during exercise is by
   a. the plasma bicarbonate reserve.
   b. muscle buffer system.
   c. red blood cells.
   d. lactate.

6. Which of the following statements about amphetamines is false?
   a. amphetamines alter the metabolism of catecholamines
   b. amphetamines increase arousal or wakefulness
   c. amphetamines redistribute blood flow to the skin and splanchnic areas
   d. amphetamines can alter receptor affinity for catecholamines

7. Which of the following statements about caffeine is false?
   a. caffeine can increase alertness and decrease drowsiness
   b. caffeine has been shown to increase lipid mobilization
   c. caffeine has been shown to increase the lactate threshold
   d. caffeine is a stimulant

8. The greatest concern over the use of smokeless tobacco is
   a. damage to teeth and gums including oral cancer.
   b. the addiction to nicotine.
   c. the development of lung cancer.
   d. the detraining effect that is caused by smokeless tobacco .

9. Blood doping could improve performance in
   a. the 100 meter sprint.
   b. the long jump.
   c. 10 mile race.
   d. 200 meter sprint.

10. Which of the following would not be caused by an overdose of cocaine?
    a. arrhythmias
    b. coma
    c. hypothermia
    d. seizures

11. Research has proven that protein supplements
    a. increase strength.
    b. increase muscle mass.
    c. increase limb circumference.
    d. None of the above.

12. Carnitine is used as a weight loss aid, the molecule is primarily involved in
    a. fatty acid transport.
    b. fatty acid oxidation.
    c. fatty acid synthesis.
    d. All of the above.

True and False

Instructions: Read each question carefully and determine if the statement is true or false. The correct answers are provided at the end of the chapter.

1. Performance improves when O_2-enriched mixtures are used at normal pressure rather than at a higher pressure than normal.

2. Breathing 100% oxygen would increase the O_2 bound to hemoglobin by 30%.

3. When breathing hyperoxic gas mixtures, the increase in the O_2 content of arterial blood is balanced by a decrease in blood flow to the working muscles such that O_2 delivery is not different from normoxic conditions.

4. Normal cross-country training increases plasma levels of naturally occurring erythropoietin.

5. Ingesting bicarbonate is believed to improve some anaerobic performances due to the enhanced ability to buffer H^+ produced during exercise.

6. Amphetamines are stimulants that have been used primarily to recover from fatigue and improve endurance.

7. The physiological benefits of the warm up would include slower enzymatic reactions at high body temperatures and a lower oxygen deficit at the onset of work.

8. A direct warm-up increases core temperature and increases arousal.

9. Increases in body temperature as a result of warm-up have been linked to improved performance.

10. Nicotine has varied effects depending on whether the parasympathetic or sympathetic nervous system is stimulated.

Matching Terms and Definitions

Instructions: Consider each term carefully and select the correct definition below. The correct answers are provided at the end of the chapter.

Terms
1. autologous transfusion
2. blood boosting/blood doping/blood packing/induced erythrocythemia
3. dental caries
4. double-blind research design
5. ergogenic aid
6. erythrocythemia
7. erythropoietin
8. homologous transfusion
9. hyperbaric chamber
10. normocythemia
11. placebo
12. sham reinfusion
13. sham withdrawal
14. sympathomimetic

Definitions

  a. Tooth decay.
  b. An inert substance that is used in experimental studies.
  c. An increase in the number of erythrocytes in the blood.
  d. Chamber where the absolute pressure is increased above atmospheric pressure.
  e. Substance that mimics the effects of epinephrine or norepinephrine, which are secreted from the sympathetic nervous system.
  f. An experimental treatment at the end of a blood doping experiment in which a needle is placed in a vein, but the subjects does not receive a reinfusion of blood.
  g. A blood transfusion using blood of the same type but from another donor.
  h. An experimental treatment at the beginning of a blood doping experiment in which a needle is placed in a vein, but blood is not withdrawn.
  i. A substance, appliance, or procedure that improves performance.
  j. Blood transfusion where the individual receives his or her own blood.
  k. Hormone that stimulates red blood cell production.
  l. Increase of the blood's hemoglobin concentration by infusion of additional red blood cells.
  m. An experimental design in which the subjects and the principal investigator are not aware of the experimental treatment order.
  n. A normal red blood cell concentration.

Answers

Multiple Choice	True and False	Terms and Definitions
1. b	1. True	1. j
2. c	2. False	2. l
3. c	3. True	3. a
4. d	4. False	4. m
5. a	5. True	5. i
6. c	6. True	6. c
7. c	7. False	7. k
8. a	8. False	8. g
9. c	9. True	9. d
10. c	10. True	10. n
11. d		11. b
12. a		12. f
		13. h
		14. e